Evangelos Koumparoudis

Medicine in the Post-consumerist Society

A Philosophical Overview

STUDIES IN MEDICAL PHILOSOPHY

Edited by Alexander Gungov and Friedrich Luft

ISSN 2367-4377

Evangelos Koumparoudis

MEDICINE IN THE
POST-CONSUMERIST SOCIETY
A Philosophical Overview

ibidem
Verlag

Bibliographic information published by the Deutsche Nationalbibliothek

Die Deutsche Nationalbibliothek lists this publication in the Deutsche Nationalbibliografie; detailed bibliographic data are available in the Internet at http://dnb.d-nb.de.

Bibliografische Information der Deutschen Nationalbibliothek

Die Deutsche Nationalbibliothek verzeichnet diese Publikation in der Deutschen Nationalbibliografie; detaillierte bibliografische Daten sind im Internet über http://dnb.d-nb.de abrufbar.

ISBN-13: 978-3-8382-1765-9

© *ibidem*-Verlag, Stuttgart 2023

Acknowledgements

I would like to express my gratitude to my dissertation supervisor, professor Alexander Gungov, for the continuous support of my PhD study and related research, for his patience, motivation, and immense knowledge. I would also like to thank deeply professor Anouk Barberousse, for her supervision during my Erasmus Scholarship from September 2019 to January 2020, in Sorbonne University. She helped me to broaden my horizons on the field of philosophy of medicine and she has been a source of enlightenment. My sincere thanks also go to professor Aneta Karageorgieva, professor Valentina Kaneva, professor Julia Vasseva Dikova and professor Zoran Dimic, for their critical comments during the first consideration of my dissertation. I am also grateful to professor Maria Dimitrova for her consultation in the philosophy of Emmanuel Levinas.

Additionally, I would like to thank professor Moses Boudourides, Vasileios Galanos, Chloe Tzia Kolyri MD, Myron Vourakis, and Stergios Aidinlis, for the discussions we have had related to the topic during all these years.

Allow me to show my heartfelt thanks to my classmates at the doctoral program in philosophy taught in English—Piotr, Francesco, Stavros, Galina and Venera—for all the good times we had, and the sharing of knowledge. Thanks also go to my classmates in Sorbonne University and the team of Philo'Doctes, Samuel, Tim, Julien, Luca, Victor, Sarah and Giada, as well as Julia Tinland.

My sincere thanks to Artemis Papachristou for the graphic editing, Paschalia Patramani, and Matthew Gill for the proofreading.

Finally, I would like to thank my family and my parents Giannis and Elena for their support and to Christine for her love, understanding and encouraging.

Table of Contents

Preface

A. Introduction

Over the last 30–40 years, digital technologies have become a considerable part of our daily life. We could not imagine ourselves not exchanging emails, short texts, and interacting on digital platforms. Furthermore, from an economic perspective, these technologies can be considered as the basic motors of production, distribution, and storage of information, the new commodity which almost substitutes for the fossil fuels and natural resources exploited massively in industrial society. This does not imply that the production and sustainability of these technologies do not demand the consumption of electricity or the fabrication of plastic, which is a product of oil refineries, or have a direct linkage with natural resources and the pollution of the environment. But if we consider that information and communication technologies gave rise to the emergence of companies like Google, Amazon, Facebook, Apple and Microsoft, known as GAFAM,[1] playing a vital role in the American and global economy, both concerning their market value, estimated in 2020 at over 4 trillion dollars,[2] and the regulatory and often biased role that they play in real politics, reaching the point where Congress was concerned enough to call for explanations from their CEOs,[3] we can understand their massive impact.

But how can we approach our computer-mediated communication and community? Is this kind of community one that retains its traditional communal characteristics? Or do digitalization, as expressed in the cyberworld, and its consequences in the real world, lead to impersonal relations? Or is something even beyond it, leading to a totally different conception of a being's identity in information society? From a broad perspective, there seem to be variable changes in our conception over

[1] Juan Carlos Miguel, Miguel Angel Casado del Rio, "GAFAnomy (Google, Amazon, Facebook and Apple): The Big Four and the b-Ecosystem," *Dynamics of Big Internet Industry Groups and Future Trends,* (2016): 127–148.

[2] J. Clemnet, "Google, Amazon, Facebook, Apple, and Microsoft (GAFAM)—statistics & facts," Statista.com, https://www.statista.com/topics/4213/google-apple-facebook-amazon-and-microsoft-gafam/, last accessed, December 20, 2020.

[3] Brian Contrearas, "Bezos, Zuckerberg and other Big Tech chiefs answer to Congress on antitrust concerns," Los Angeles Times, July 29, 2020,https://www.latimes.com/politics/story/2020-07-29/congress-to-grill-tech-industry-chiefs, last accessed, December 20,2020.

space and time. David Harvey, in his *The Condition of Postmodernity* (1989), speaks about such a time-space compression, the revolutionary processes brought about by technology that modify the objective qualities of space and time, and—consequently—the way we represent the world to ourselves.[4] From another perspective, Zygmunt Bauman, in his *Liquid Modernity* (2000), describes the passage from **"hard" and "solid"** to liquid modernity, from the society of solid and heavy machinery to the lightness of an email. But this does not only have to do with the means of production; people live in uncertainty and perceive time as an objective instantaneity. People act faster and move faster; their conception of time is under the domination of individuality, which always seeks ways to escape. This differential access to instantaneity is equal to such an unpredictability connected by the new social status with freedom, something peculiar for example in the feudal society since the workers were stuck in immobility in the courts of their landlords.[5]

Bauman also states that in the society of producers, health was set as a standard; in the society of consumers,[6] the ideal is fitness. They may have a synonymous use as they relate to the care of the body, but they are different to a certain extent. Health in the society of producers was a normative concept, which was related to endurance—a general well-being with easily measurable parameters so that the social role of the producers could be achieved—and this was the capacity to work in the factory, to perform heavy tasks, etc. In our consumer society, fitness becomes like any other concept—anything but solid; there is no real criterion to define fitness. It is something that lies in the future and is connected with the adaptability and flexibility of the body. It should always be seen as something in excess, ready to meet the extraordinary, that which is not mundane. If health is something normative, fitness is the breaking of all norms. Fitness has no real end; it concerns a momentary satisfaction of reaching a goal in the breaks between hard-working days. But as normative as health can be, in the age of liquid modernity it is even more fragile. What yesterday was considered normal today could be worrying or pathological.[7] New states of the body can be taken as reasons for medical intervention. In this case, we should consider not only states that may facilitate life—for example, a hip-replacement oper-

4   David Harvey, *The Condition of Postmodernity* (New Jersey: Wiley-Blackwell, 1989), 241.
5   Zygmunt Bauman, *Liquid Modernity* (London: Polity Press, 2000), 120–121.
6   Bauman introduced the term in his *Life in Fragments* (Polity Press, 1996).
7   Zygmunt Bauman, *Liquid Modernity*, 79.

ation—but, more importantly, the medical interventions biased by the dominant beauty standards promoted massively through mass and social media, like plastic surgeries and interventions of weight loss without a serious reason, such as diabetes or cardiovascular problems. The definition of disease also becomes quite blurred. It is not something with a start and end, but always implies an awareness of being healthy, something grasped by the existence of all kinds of healthy diets, nutrient supplements, etc. At this point, we could also account for ideas that may have a political or ecological signification, like veganism, the non-consumption of meat and dairy products, or even herbalism, the consumption of herbs rather than chemically manufactured drugs (although most of them could be conceived of as beneficial supplements). Bauman ends with the assumption that health tends to be similar to the instability of fitness, generating uncertainty and anxiety.

This instantaneity of time and space, from another perspective, can be linked with an urge of instantaneity in decision-making. This decision-making, however, today, in some cases, is based on algorithmic automation. Algorithms in a broad sense are encoded procedures for transforming input data into the desired output, based on specific calculations. The procedures name both a problem and the steps by which it should be solved.[8] In general, they seek to create patterns based on certain causation and correlation; they also have capacities of adaptability which are "machine learning" techniques, something that will be analyzed extensively in our fifth chapter. These algorithms are used, for example, in spelling correction, fraud prevention, risk analysis, and medical science. To this very introductory point, we only question how human rights and dignity can be safeguarded by these technologies. Are there any racial, ethnic, or gender biases more or less likely in these systems? Is there a chance through a process of automated (or semi-automated) profile categorization for a person to be excluded from health insurance or employment, or even be regarded as a criminal?

Rafael Capurro describes some aspects of medicine in this kind of information-based society.[9] One basic element is how information over-

---

[8]   Gillespie Tarleton, "The Relevance of Algorithms," in *Media technologies: Essays on communication, materiality, and society*, ed. by T. Gillespie, P. J. Boczkowski, and K. A. Foot (Cambridge, Mass.: MIT Press, 2014), 167–94.

[9]   Rafael Capurro, "Medicine in the Information Society and Knowledge," Keynote at the European Summit for Clinical Nanomedicine and Targeted Medicine (CLINAM), Basel, Switzerland, June 23–26, 2013, http://www.capurro.de/Medicine2_0.html, last accessed, December 20, 2020.

load affects physicians and patients with the large amounts of information that are generated by medical research and experimentation, which is linked today to what is called Evidence-Based Medicine. This may lead to possible disorientation or reshaping the role of the doctor from someone who knows to someone whose knowledge is under consideration by a well-informed patient. Secondly, he focuses on the interactivity between doctors and digital native patients, as in the possible attribution of negligence to a hospital that does not provide digital information-based interaction—for instance, information on patients' conditions and recovery processes. He also points out issues of privacy, as in what manner personal data will be used, its security and safety, and its use for a maleficent reason or with poor consequences. Furthermore, he strives towards the implications of new technologies on personalized medicine and the possibility of computer-mediated systems of communication to regulate the doctor-patient relationship, consequently reducing patients' autonomy and excluding, for example, elder patients. Finally, he speaks about the possible transformation of the "corpus", from "Habeas Corpus", into "Habeas Data". This is a relatively good briefing on some of the changes, but what else should we consider in our approach?

B. The Goal and Objectives

What is the general goal of this book? It is to point out, from a philosophical perspective, certain aspects of medical practices correlated to the spectrum of biological and social sciences, in a society that we have called post-consumerist. First, we have to define the society characterized by high technology and digitalized infrastructure and called post-consumerist. We will describe the changes revolving around the new conception of commodity, the forms of its unconditional investment without equivalences, the symbolic dimension it may take, and how it is reproduced in a manner leading to economic speculation. Second, we describe the changes in the perception of time and space, how, on the one hand, time is compressed and the subject is submerged into instantaneity, and, on the other, everything becomes liquid. Additionally, the new status of being's identity in the post-consumerist society is given in our analysis of the term **trace** and how it is involved in **impersonal personality** relations, used as **an abstract statistical unit** in various forms of **conversions (real-semblances),** which can remain real for all practical purposes. This kind of society not only produces and distributes information but also various forms of disinformation spread by the elites, aiming at manipulation. Therefore, we will try to reveal these mechanisms, mainly through the way meaning and sense are produced, how intersubjective relations change, and how proximity, real-semblance, and trace dramatize a central role in the mechanisms of disinformation. Furthermore, we consider if an alternative could be proposed based on such an intersubjective relation which can surpass the dominant signification as posed by the elites, placing the correct or normative field of authority, through a process of mutual glaring. How is computational neuroscience related to artificial intelligence? What is the role of neuron mirrors and is there a possible relation with phenomenology? In which ways does being attain exteriority? Are there changes in the forms of medical reasoning? What are the roles of the doctor and patient today? Does the doctor base his diagnosis and treatment in a strictly objective way, conceiving of the patient as a diseased body, or are there models that propose that the doctor should also have knowledge of the subjective experience of the patient? How do they feel? How do their lives change in relation to their environment, their family? How are the social and cultural beliefs that they may have involved in the doctor-patient relationship? Do all these questions have to do with problems and puzzles? Thus, can we speak about paradigmatic changes in medicine (and medical philosophy)? What happens with knowledge acquisition after the explosion of Big Data? How does it apply to medicine and is it efficient? When it comes to epistemology, what are Big Data's limits? Can correlation replace the usual hypothetico-deductive medical reasoning? And lastly, is it efficient or should we reconsider reasoning by taking into account pragmatics and abduction? Is there any need for interdisciplinarity between sciences, since Big Data, in some cases, concerns more than one field? How do we approach the categorization of diseases today? What are the definitions of health and disease after George Canguilhem and the debate of normativism and naturalism?

What are the changes that information society has brought to our embodiment if we consider the various forms of virtual reality and cyberenvironments? Are there new forms of control over the body after the rise of these technologies, reconstructing the traditional notions of citizens, reducing them to a form of bare life? What happens with prosthetics, organ transplantation, and 3D-printed biomaterials? How do they affect our relationship with our bodies, and do they challenge the role of medicine? How do the new theories of post-humanism and transhumanism shape a fusion of machine and organism and how the binarity of natural systems altered? Could we visualize a new stage of evolution, in which humans in their fusion with machines will defeat death and come to increasingly dominate nature?

C. Methodology and Chapter Structure

We will try to give answers to all these questions by following political philosophy—mainly that of Jean-François Lyotard and his theory of libidinal economy and the postmodern condition; Jean Baudrillard and his theory of simulation; Zygmunt Bauman in his conceptions of consumerism; and Alexander Gungov with his notion of real-semblance in Chapter 1. Phenomenology and hermeneutics will help us clarify the way meaning and sense is produced in the post-consumerist society, just as post-structuralism will be used to describe the mechanisms of manipulation in Chapter 2. In Chapter 3, theories of neuroscience will be seen in relation with artificial intelligence and classical phenomenology; also, we will proceed to certain formalizations through which being can attain exteriority. In Chapter 4, the theory of Thomas Kuhn will help us see how medicine (and the philosophy of medicine) itself poses problems, creates puzzles, and can make paradigmatic shifts; this will be done by presenting the two models of medical reasoning: the biomedical or objective, and the humanistic or subjective. In Chapter 5, we will refer to more technical issues like the various mathematical models by which the creation and management of Big Data are achieved; specific research in medicine will illuminate its applications and limits. The categorization of disease (taxonomy) will be presented through a historical prism and, also, we will refer to the need for categorization on a molecular basis. The idea of the patient's safety will be exposed in relation to Gungov's theory and the interdisciplinarity between sciences via the theory of Anne-Françoise Schmid and Muriel Mambrini-Doudet. The relations between doctor and patient will be approached through Emmanuel Levinas and Jacques Derrida as well as through our basic assumptions. In the final chapter 6, the idea of new forms of embodiment will be seen according to political philosophy, phenomenology, and ideas belonging to the posthumanist and transhumanist tradition.

In the first section, Chapter 1 **(Post-consumption)**, we try to give a general overview of the transition from the society of producers to the society of consumers, examining some characteristics of consumerism as approached mainly by Lyotard, Baudrillard, and Bauman, and the move to a post-consumerist society, as defined by Gungov. Then, with the help of aesthetics (theory of cinema), we formulate what we will call **trace,** as substituting a being's identity, in the second section. Very briefly, what are these aspects? In the theory of Lyotard, we emphasize the role that libido plays in the unconditional investment of capital, as the (post)consumption of desired-desires, leaving aside the general equivalences that can be utilized as a measure for the value of commodities. We also see that the postmodern world cannot subscribe to the great narratives of the modern era; he also proclaims the role that digitalization of society comes to play nowadays. Baudrillard, on the other hand, focuses his attention on the consumption of signs and messages, rather than commodities, through a general code of signification run by the system. In his early considerations, he exemplifies these commodities as simulations, as pseudo-objects which may have an over-abundance of signs but do not signify anything; he also speaks for simulations in our social relations, which in some cases are always mediated and fake, as in advertising. In his later works, he expands the symbolic dimension of exchangeability, as the exchangeability of work, commodities, strikes, and even death. The general signification of the code absorbs everything, turning the society into a factory and placing the subject between a given reality and an upper realm of hyperreality. Bauman speaks about a society in which the consumer himself becomes a commodity. He also speaks about a liquid life which reduces everything to the sphere of **nowness**, of an infinite succession of presents. Finally, it is important to mention his definitions of underclass or outcasts as the people living on the margin of society who could be perfect candidates for statistical reasons. Gungov starts from this category of marginalized citizens to reformulate them into statistical units as the actors of various converted forms (a kind of real semblances that can remain real for all practical purposes), like the privatization of public property (investors), civil protests (protestors), elections (voters), and financial crises (taxpayers, mortgage payers). In the second section, we reveal the existence of a real-sembling identity of the statistical units shaped in the post-consumerist society encapsulated by the term **trace**. The subject—from an impersonal personality placed somewhere in the big malls of late consumerist society possibly capable of ascribing a meaning to his being, or conceive otherness—is transformed into a disposable personal impersonality, consuming personally-targeted advertisements of products and services through digital platforms, but for impersonal speculation, lost in a non-linear matrix of cyberspace, and most importantly, in the horizon of "now".

In the second chapter **(Ethics, Meaning, and Sense in the Post-Consumerist Society)**, we seek to explore how meaning and sense are produced in the post-consumerist society. We pass from a classical phenomenological and hermeneutical analysis, to an attempt to better understand issues like the perception of time, history, tradition, understanding, language, and the Other, to end up with a modified structural analysis incorporating elements of speculative philosophy to uncover the methods through which manipulation or disinformation is spread by the elites so they can impose their dominance upon the statistical units, as well as to propose an alternative. To summarize how this is achieved, it all has to do with the relationship between those who belong to the center (elites, corporations, banks, etc.) and those who belong to the periphery (statistical units), in the horizon of "now". This two-sided relation is formulated by three parameters: proximity, real-semblance, and trace. The parameter that is not shared between those two is proximity; through the non-proximal relation the domination is achieved, but as we will see it is a perplexing scheme that cannot be summarized in two lines. Then we introduce some terms, like the performativity of the action and avulsion. The first is important from an ethical, or better axiological, perspective; it refers to the decentered subject (described by structuralism onwards) and its participation in discourse or speech acts, and therefore its mediated formation of identity (that may contain social, political, and religious discourses); the second refers to a phenomenon in which in a topological space of representations, like a news feed of an application, has feedback that functions in such a manner that the production of its meaning brings an a priori stable beyond every contextualization. We then proceed with the description of what we call "mutual glaring" as a form of intersubjective "mutual understanding", beyond the maxim of signification of the center or the elites. Finally, we close by proposing an alternative that is based on the notions of arbitrariness and the Hegelian topsy-turvy world.

In the third chapter **(Self-Portrait in a Neuron Mirror)**, we first deal with computational neuroscience, a project that started in the late 1980s and has continued up to our day. It is an overall attempt to describe human brain function through networks of neurons. It is important to see this neuro-reductivist approach in relation to its fusion with artificial intelligence programs, known as connectionist. The connectionists created algorithms called "neuron networks" capable of imitating human imagination. Against the reductionism that computational neuroscience proposes, we briefly expose an alternative, which is the discovery of the mirror neurons in macaque monkeys in the late '80s and the existence of human analogues via indirect ways such as MRI, fMRI, PET scan, etc. This neuroscientific model can be seen as a fundamental mechanism of grasping the actions of others, as well as their emotions, and also participates in the process of learning; thus, the relation from merely subjective, as in computational neuroscience, turns intersubjective and also intentional as we open to the world and others. These findings help us to understand our intersubjective aspirations of the second chapter, defined as "mutual glaring" or "mutual understanding". We illuminate them further with various phenomenological approaches—mainly those of Edmund Husserl and his theories of intentionality and empathy; Max Scheler and his accounts on the feelings of others and the role that they play in our experiencing of others; and the theory of embodied cognition by Maurice Merleau-Ponty, and, finally, Hans-Georg Gadamer. As for the second possible imitation of human imagination, we refer to speculative poetics with a major poem of postmodernity, John Ashbery's "Self-Portrait in a Convex Mirror", and poetry as well as poetics as a possible distinctive characteristic of human imagination. Finally, we pass even beyond the spheres of psychoanalysis and metaphysics by describing cases in which being is enclosed (restrictive formalizations of Dehors) and its attempts to attain exteriority.

In the fourth chapter **(Objective and Subjective Medical Reasoning: A Philosophical Overview)**, we investigate how the philosophy of medicine (and medicine itself), creates puzzles, poses problems, and creates paradigms, following the analysis of Thomas Kuhn, to enrich the debate that has arisen over the last years and revolves around the question as to if the philosophy of medicine can be a separate field. We compare the two forms of medical reasoning—biomedical, or objective, and human-based, or subjective—to clarify these considerations. The first concerns the dominant biomedicine, which has as its central focus, substance matter and is therefore connected with materialism or physicalism, as well as a metaphysical presupposition—reductionism. For the second, holism or dualism is its metaphysical grounding and its metaphysical presupposition is emergentism. The first conceives of the body as a diseased entity from which the doctor should obtain objective clinical data in order to proceed to diagnosis, treatment, and prognosis, while the second focuses more on the subjective experience of the illness by the patient and the interaction with his environment, social, working, religious, etc. The models of objective medical reasoning can be based on

Bayesian analysis (when we have to predict a future event), or on frequentist statistics (when, for example, we seek the frequency of a symptom, disease, etc.) The objectivity can also be grasped through what has been called Evidence-Based Medicine, calling for more reliance on evidence obtained from current published research and randomized control trials. As for models of subjective thinking, we put forward the models proposed by Eric Cassel, whose view is somewhere between subjectivity and objectivity in reasoning, the biopsychosocial model of George L. Engel, who proposes the correction of the biomedical model on three levels (recognition of complex causation, recognition of various levels of activity, and recognition of the individual variability of disease), the infomedical model of Laurence Foss, in which information has a leading role, and—finally—the narrative model, in which the patient unfolds his personal experience in a form of storytelling.

In the fifth chapter **(The Impact of Big Data on Medicine)**, we emphasize the role of Big Data as generated in the domain of health in biological sciences. We see how it changed our medical approach and contributed to precision medicine and integrative biology. We present the methods of data analysis such as data mining, machine learning, and deep learning for their application in medicine by presenting certain research. We also uncover epistemological problems, such as how knowledge can be acquired through it, and what its efficacy and limits are. We then explore the role of the internet 2.0 in medical practice; we present the benefits for doctors, such as easier access to medical databases, and patients, such as medical information acquired and a possible active role, as well as the dangers and the major disadvantages, such as biased medical information. We then proceed to a historical overview of the taxonomy of the various diseases in order to later expose the need for categorization on a molecular basis. The limits of Big Data and Randomized Control Trials will also be analyzed, when, for example, we pass from Big Data to Smart Data; as for the RCTs, which are considered the gold standard for medical research, we can give examples of prior knowledge they may demand and the role of various policymakers. We then strive towards the obscure empiricism of Big Data, claiming that correlation is enough, and we will also reconsider if reasoning can be data-driven or hypothesis-driven, implementing hypothetico-deductive medical reasoning in comparison with Gungov's interpretation of abductive method in his *Patient's Safety: The Relevance of Logic in Medical Care* and the generic conception of epistemology as posed by Schmid and Mambrini-Doudet. We will also reconsider the patient-doctor relationship and medical decision-making through the prism of Emmanuel Levinas and Jacques Derrida, as well as some of our basic assumptions throughout this book, such as glaring. Finally, we focus on the debate about naturalism and normativism in the conception of illness and disease.

The final, sixth chapter **(Information Society and a New Form of Embodiment)** aims to present the various changes in our embodying experience shaped by the new information, virtual, and robotic technologies, as well as their political and moral effect. The essay is also expanded to encapsulate the new conceptions in our approach to bodily transformation, medicine, and sexuality, strongly interconnected with the above facts. Our analysis is structured according to six different categories of embodiment: bodies, bodily governance, transforming bodies, virtual bodies, medical bodies, and·sexual bodies. The political impact is mainly given through the description of the forms of bodily governance, like personal and biometric data collection used for massive surveillance and as a measure for defining the "ideal" standards of our social life. The possibilities provided by classical and 3D-printed organ transplantation and the use of prosthetic and cosmetic surgeries led us to rethink our bodies as transforming or as being in a process of becoming. Our immersion in virtual environments and the use of avatars raise questions about embodying and disembodying experiences and the formation of our identities in the virtual world. The dominant biomedical model seems to be challenged by more human-based approaches emphasizing the subjective narratives of the patient, consequently contributing to the more ethical and non-normative treatment of people with special needs and elder people. Furthermore, the use of robotics in the care of people with mobility or mental problems brings dilemmas in the human-machine interaction and the roles of caregivers, care receivers, and robots. Additionally, after structuralism and post-structuralism, the natural-binary systems have been thoroughly criticized; this fact gave birth to feminist theories which consider that gender is socially constructed and that the body, and therefore the gendered body, is a disembodied prosthesis of information or a fusion between machine and organism. Finally, information technologies and progress in medicine and biotechnology can be seen as a chance to surpass the limits of our humanity, defeat death, and give a totally different perspective on our evolution, cognition, and embodiment, and this is shaped by various theories on transhumanism.

Chapter 1:
Post-Consumption

1.1 Introduction: Towards Aspects of Post-Consumerism

What distinguishes the age in which mass production was the main dogma of the economy, characterized by heavy machinery, with its capital-intensive technologies, and the social formation shaped by relatively static structures such as the factory (Fordist model), from our current post-industrial society, in which high technology and information knowledge play a vital role? As we will see, mass consumption gradually supersedes mass production and the commodity (if we follow classical political economy). Although it retains part of its use-value and circulation, it seems that its reproduction and symbolic exchange-value now pass to a sphere that can be called "surplus value from the periphery". Beyond the broad image we also have to look upon the subject of this post-industrial information society, which we will call post-consumerist. Is the subject of post-consumerist society only an addict of mass consumption, or something more? What are the roles of desire, libido, and death, as some of the main aspects of the passage from the consumerist society to post-consumerist? Are there broad categories of citizens in both of them? In order to give answers to all these questions, briefly posed above, we will examine the theories of Jean-Francois Lyotard, mainly in *Libidinal Economy* (1974) and *The Postmodern Condition* (1979), Jean Baudrillard and his analysis of *Consumer Society* (1970) and *Symbolic Exchange and Death* (1976) and more of what he calls **hyperreality and simulation**, Zygmunt Bayman and his *Consuming Life* (2007), and finally Alexander Gungov and his theory about post-consumerist society and **real-semblance**. We will deal with the latter, real-semblance, in depth not only in this first introductory chapter but also in the second, and partially throughout this book.

Lyotard's *Libidinal Economy* (1974) should be seen as a book written in the aftermath of the uprising in May 1968 in France. It is an attempt to fuse classical notions of Freudian psychoanalysis with the Marxist tradition and simultaneously to break the bonds with it by seeking new forces within society like **libidinal energy**. It communicates with radical and revolutionary writings of its age like *Capitalism and Schizophrenia* (1972) by Gilles Deleuze and Felix Guattari, as well as the

writings of Baudrillard and Pierre Klossowski. It is a relatively difficult
book both for its content and style of writing, both of which belong to the
early Lyotard—the so-called libidinal phase. But what should we take
from this book in relation to the questions that we have posed? We will
stick more to the more applied aspects of the book, and not, for example,
to the way libidinal energies (libidinal intensities, following Freud's primary processes of unconscious and affects, like feelings, and desires;
Lyotard mainly focuses on sexual desire) are created and diffused in the
society, such as the Libidinal band, the bar, the Great Zero.[10] Lyotard
introduces the term **simulacrum/exorbitant** as something exchangeable
or equivalent (he follows St. Augustine's idea of simulacra, as the generalized equivalence expressed by the unity of God, and he responds to
Pierre Klossowski's analysis of "Living Currency"). In capitalism, the
rule of the value of goods is based on certain equivalences and assures
the exchangeability between money and goods, but there are some cases
in which this rule is not implemented. In the libidinal economy, the libido invests unconditionally; for example, in prostitution, the exchange is
realized between the desire of the prostitute and a desire of capital's
demand to profit from the prostitute's body.[11] Libidinal exchanges are
exorbitant; there is no equivalent or forms of accountability. Every exchange of this form, through the metamorphosis and polysemous character of the libido, looks for such a sacrifice so the most exorbitant price
will be achieved. Consequently, we meet a form of speculation without
equivalences, even without real products. It is only the desire which is
invested, reproduced, and of course, consumed. Can this consumption of
phantasms as products of our desire be compatible with an idea of post-
consumption? Of course, yes, since we consume a desired-desire, which
stands on its own, driven by libido.

In his *The Postmodern Condition* (1979), probably his most well-
known book and determining the transition from modernity to post-

---

[10]   Jean François Lyotard, *Libidinal Economy*, trans. Iain Hamilton Grant (Indianapolis:
Indiana University Press, 1993), 1118.

[11]   "As soon as one admits the inexchangeability of phantasms, one must accept decisive-
ly the necessity of the conservation of political economy and capital. Since it results
from this inexchangeability that they are inevitably substituted by doubles or simulacra, and therefore that libidinal 'riches' are misrepresented in the economic signs of
this wealth which they represent but which, also, will forever differ from them in
terms of consumption... is this libidinal economy; a political economy without a be-
trayed or alienated 'origin', without a theory of value. A currency therefore in the
sense of Roman paganism and theatrical theology admitting only tensor signs, only
masks hiding no face, only surfaces without a back stage, only prices without values"
Ibid., 92–93.

modernity, Lyotard claims that in the postmodern world it has become difficult to subscribe to the great narratives which previously conditioned existence. These narratives were, for example, forms of salvation as expressed in various religions, or proclaimed the emancipation of the masses; a typical example is Marxist theory, or therapy, if we consider the Freudian psychoanalytical revolution and its impact. Postmodernism can be approached in terms of an anti-foundationalism, more as a mood rather than as a period. A pragmatic and experimentalist attitude defines its subject matter. There are two main theoretical aspects—first, event, and second, justice. An event occurs when it happens, without having any specific identity. The identification of what happened can only happen when the event is inserted into a determined structure through which it will signal meaning to the happening. Lyotard continues his analysis on anti-foundationalism by saying that knowledge is not accumulated in libraries and museums, but increasingly in our time is stored in less material forms like microchips and computer disks. Therefore, knowledge cannot be hierarchized and obtain a certain significance. Furthermore, any foundational theory homogenizes rather than reveals the particularity of singular events, leaving no place for genuine thinking.[12] The postmodern society always strives towards the great narratives of modernity and the digitalization of society in which knowledge and scientific know-how is reduced to the will and patents of corporations. The struggle of nation-states for natural resources in the past now turns to the information commodity as stored information. The huge multinationals which can more efficiently deal with these volumes of information will gradually take over the sovereignty of the nation-state.[13] If we consider that the book was written 40 years ago, Lyotard was able to visualize our current form of society in which the utopia of Silicon Valley as the Mecca of information technologies seems to be one of the major centers of economic wealth and power, in some cases bypassing regulations and privacy, if we consider, for example, the Cambridge Analytica scandal.[14] Finally. justice has a specific sense in his philosophy. Justice should be more like an "event". After the metanarrative theory, there are various

---

[12]   Thomas Docherty, "Postmodernist Theory", in *Twentieth-Century Continental Philosophy*, ed. Richard Kearny (London: Routledge, 1994), 397.

[13]   Peter Gratton, "Jean François Lyotar", *The Stanford Encyclopedia of Philosophy* (Winter 2018 Edition), Edward N. Zalta, ed., URL = <https://plato.stanford.edu/archives/win2018/entries/lyotard/>.

[14]   "The Cambridge Analytica Files", The Guardian, https://www.theguardian.com/news/series/cambridge-analytica-files. last accessed, December 20, 2020.

grounds that we base our judgments on in aesthetic, ethical, and political language-games. Consequently, our judgments turn to simple conditions of living, without certain criteria.

If we focus on Baudrillard's *The Consumer Society* (1970), although it is a book devoted to consumerism, certain aspects can be considered as post-consumption. Baudrillard says that our consumption is no longer consumption of commodities; rather, we consume signs (messages and images). Subsequently, the consumer should have a capacity of interpretation of the system of consumption to know what to consume. There is a code which gives meaning to the commodities (signification), so commodities do not hold their use-value anymore, but are characterized by what they signify. Their signification does not shape what they do, but shows their relationship to the entire system of commodities and signs. Furthermore, the system promotes individual differentiation or personalization; individuals constantly seek how to distinguish themselves from others. According to Baudrillard, this is not a matter of personal choice; it is the code of the system that makes individuals both similar and different. Therefore, we should proceed from a conception of conscious social dynamics to the unconscious social logic of signs and the code. He then makes a distinction between those who have a mastery over the code, which are the upper classes, while the middle and lower classes lack this mastery of the code and tend to fetishize objects, seeking to prove themselves and find salvation through them. An idea which is central in this book is that of simulations; this idea is broadened in his *Symbolic Exchange and Death* (1976). Simulations are defined first as sham objects, and these objects define our consumer society. They are objects that offer an abundance of signs that they are real, but actually, they are not. He gives the examples of kitsch, trashy objects, and souvenirs as objects that have a superabundance of signs but no real signification. They are pseudo-objects of imitation and reproduction. The way we are exposed to mass media and mass advertising is also a form of simulation, a form of simulated social relations. They claim to have an intimacy which is always fake and mediated; they just reproduce elements of the code. Furthermore, by consuming advertisements we are submitted to post-consumption since we consume the simulation of the object sold.[15]

Baudrillard, in his *Symbolic Exchange and Death* (1976), borrows the idea of symbolic exchange of goods in primitive societies (Mauss's

---

[15]   Jean Baudrillard, *The Consumer Society, Myths and Structures*, (London: Sage, 1998), 1–24.

anthropological analysis of the Gift) and he expands it to the late consumerist society, through a passage from a classical Marxist perspective, and through psychoanalysis—mainly from Sigmund Freud and Jacques Lacan. Baudrillard claims that the current forms of exchange of commodities do not follow the law of value, but a structural law of value; this structural law has no reference to a dominant class or relation of forces.[16] There are also changes in the form of labor; there is no more proper signification of a particular type of labor, but only a system where jobs are exchanged.[17] We no longer work, but we perform acts of production. The workers are not agents of exploitation, but rather are characterized by their mobility and exchangeability.[18] There is a general code of signification (broader than that of the *Consumer Society*, which is centered on commodities) run by the system which absorbs and gives a symbolic value to everything, from labor to commodities, strikes, and even death. This code always stands between a real given realm (a reality principle) and a symbolic dimension which is also apparent forming a hyperreality. The subjects of the consumerist society are always participants in this process of simulation between the two realities. The simulation today gives these attributes to the commodity, and its function adopts only its exchange value to hide the fact that it circulates like a sign and reproduces the code.[19] Today there is only reproductive labor as well as reproductive consumption.[20] Our childhood, our daily habits, our relationships, and our unconscious drives are integrated into this general code; consequently, our personal choice of work, which sometimes seems to be tailor-made, signifies that the **die is cast**; as a result the absorption will be total.[21] The factory of the Fordist model now moves to the whole society; society now becomes a factory-society. The equivalence of wage and labor power presupposes the death of the worker, as the commodity presupposes the symbolic extermination of the object. However, this death is not differentiated from a general free time and fulfillment of life, but rather is a form of a slow death from gradual exhaustion as opposed to a violent death.[22] Wages are the mark of a poisonous gift, which epitomizes the whole code and the dominant social relation.

---

[16] Jean Baudrillard, *Symbolic Exchange and Death,* trans. Iain Hamilton Grant (London: Sage, 1993), 10.
[17] Ibid., 13.
[18] Ibid., 18.
[19] Ibid., 31.
[20] Ibid., 28.
[21] Ibid., 14.
[22] Ibid., 39.

Bauman, in his *Consuming Life* (2007), describes three major cases that can characterize the consumerist society. The first concerns the rise of social networking sites as networks of social cyber-interaction in which social life is substituted by a cyber-life. In these sites, users choose to share and expose moments of their lives, both recreational and working. Bauman also describes the existence of dating sites in which flirting via face-to-face interaction is deferred and the users attempt to find a perfect match through the exhaustive profiles of their possible partners. The second refers to the new computerized systems of corporations which categorize callers (and users) depending on their value (purchasing capacity, the balance of their bank accounts). Although this could be a technology that increases the efficiency of their function, the real purpose is that they work as a machine that filters out the so-called flawed consumers. The third describes the case of a young woman from New Zealand (with a master's degree) who was trying to find a job in the UK; selective immigration policies set the condition for her entry to the UK as the submission of a certification that she already had been awarded by a corporation, having passing certain qualification tests,.[23]

With these three cases, he points out that everyone is nudged to promote an attractive commodity in the market; this commodity is themselves. They become both the promoters and the commodity they promote. The subjectivity of the subject is forced to become and remain a sellable commodity. In the consumerist society, we have a transition from commodity fetishism to subjectivity fetishism.[24] One of the major themes is that the society of producers became a society of consumers. The society of producers was a society that placed emphasis on durability and long-term security.[25] In the consumerist society, everything becomes liquid. There is instability of desires and needs, an instant urge for consumption, and instant disposal of objects; it is all about speed, excess, and waste, and our perception of time becomes instantaneous. Life is today a succession of presents, a collection of instants with varying intensity. It is a life of **nowness**, that would not allow a second chance, or delay.[26] In the society of producers the body would be a worker or soldier. The society of producers dominated bodies, so they could be placed in their natural habitat, the factory or the battlefield. In the society of

---

[23]   Zygmunt Bauman, *Consuming Life*, 1–6.
[24]   Ibid., 14.
[25]   Ibid., 31.
[26]   Ibid., 35.

consumers, people focus from an early age on the management of their spirit, and the practice of the body becomes an individual task.[27]

It is important to mention Bauman's conception of the **underclass**, or **outcast**, which will help us to follow Gungov's thought (the term **statistical units**), as well as our analysis, revolving around the passage from identity to trace. The underclass in a manner has associations with the underworld. It refers to poor people who drop out of school, young mothers without the benefit of marriage who go on welfare, homeless people, beggars, immigrants without official papers, and even teenage gang members.[28]The social state tends to homogenize all these abstract social groups since all of them could appeal to a welfare system, a source of solidarity which can recycle society into a common good, but avoiding the collateral damage of the extremes of misery and indignity. This misery and indignity are the fear of passing to the category of the excluded of **human waste**.[29]

Gungov, in his "Real Semblance Flourishing in Post-Consumerist Society",[30] focuses on the function of converted forms, a notion introduced by Karl Marx. These forms are a kind of real-semblance, a semblance in relation with genuine reality, which can remain real for all practical proposes. It is distinguished from the Hegelian sublation in which illusion is gradually overcome and reaches an absolute truth. It is also different from the simulation of Baudrillard in which the simulation hides the reality and is transferred to the realm of hyperreality. It can be exemplified in a saying like: "the surface gloss of good manners"; here the two levels of reality, the one real and the other fake, preserve their particular significance. Converted forms are forms of alienation of human relations turned into a fetish. The most common are commodity value and capital. The first has for the illusion that its value is formed due to exchange value, but, in reality, it depends on universal abstract labor to produce a commodity, while capital, the source of profit, is based on surplus labor hours and not something enigmatic. Gungov, following Bauman, as analyzed just above, claims that the consumers who sell themselves are also converted. But the determining element in our analysis is what happens to the underclass. The underclass is a perfect candidate to become an **abstract statistical unit** and adopt a statisti-

---

27   Ibid., 54.
28   Ibid., 134.
29   Ibid., 144.
30   Cf. Alexander Gungov, "Real Semblance Flourishing in Post-Consumerist Society", *Sofia Philosophical Review*, vol. VII, No. 2, 2013.

cal value. These statistical units participate in at least four categories of
social interaction where the converted forms enter deeper layers of genuine reality. These four categories are mass privatization, elections, civil
protests, and financial crises. As for the first category, the statistical units
play the role of **investors**. The major example provided by Gungov is
what happened after the fall of formerly socialist states. The problem of
how formerly state property could pass to the hands of private interests
could be solved by printing voucher books. Everyone was welcome to
buy assets. In the case that no one could be bothered to buy (from the
people having no real funds up to economically powerful hedge funds)
this transformation could never happen. So, state property is converted to
private though the intermediation of these units. In the case of elections,
the statistical units are transformed into **voters**. If no one votes then the
entire representative system will collapse. It does not matter if they are
conservative or progressive, etc.; candidates will be elected and the par-
ties that participate in the elections, if they reach a certain limit, will be
financially rewarded. Statistical units can also transform into **protestors.**
Gungov gives the examples of the 2011 Middle East Spring, Kiev 2013,
etc. The protestors, although they claim to be the avant-garde of civil
movement, never reach a Hegelian absolute knowing; they can just be
part of the next social embodiment, an overthrow of a government, the
formation of a new one, etc. Statistical units as **protestors** just keep the
show going. According to Gungov, the most enigmatic role of statistical
units is in financial crises. Giving the example of Iceland, which, after
the bankruptcy of its banking system, resisted implementing austerity
measures and heavy taxation of the citizens to repay state loans and en-
tered the downward spiral of debt repayment, Gungov asserts that the
Icelandic people indirectly indicated the most fundamental element of
post-consumerism, economic speculation. The converted social relation
in which financial speculation rests is the infinite possibilities of the
transformation of statistical units. In the opposite direction, statistical
units, such as **taxpayers** and **mortgage payers**, are a form of dead souls
in resurrection, which remain unsellable but can be used for practical
purposes, such as statistical fiscal correction, like the workers in the
society of producers, utilized as means for the increase of the available
values. (Post)consumers are now the means of an infinite commercial
exchange forming a Gross Domestic Product.

1.2 From Identity to Trace

Our analysis starts from the Wong Kar-wai film *Chungking Express*. This starting point is not random, and—as will be shown—this film is not only remarkable because of its pioneering techniques in filmmaking, but in our opinion, it introduces notable notions to our way of understanding being in its transition, [31] in its transition, from the late consumerist society to the post-consumerist society.[32]

If we were to speak about the notion of time in the works of Wong Kar-wai, one word could possibly describe its essence: **co-presence**. This is fully epitomized in his *Chungking Express*, but in a way had been cultivated in his earlier cinematography. The significant shift made in this movie concerning the narrative techniques is not the non-linearity of the main plot but this strange **co-presence of time**. [33] All the possible **co-presenting** layers of time are discrete and are given straightforwardly to the spectator. The general narrative time is interwoven with an intermediate time in most cases. But how does Wong achieve this, and more prominently, for the first time in movie history? He uses a mixture of slow motion, fast forward, and freeze-frame, mainly in the editing of the movie.[34] More precisely, *Chungking Express* is filmed in the metropolis of Hong Kong, with its daily frenzied pace of life. The scenery, for example, the moving crowd or the neon lights of a large boulevard, are usually shown with fast-forward speed, but at the same time, the main characters are filmed in parallel, with slow motion speed, even freeze-frame, and mainly with close-up shots. With this kind of "illusion", or as we call it, **co-presence of time**, the director emphasizes the perception of subjective time through the actions of the main characters of the movie. Simultaneously, he emphasizes the intersubjective perception of time, occurring from the interaction of the main characters, with the objectivity of the frenzied time of Hong Kong. Thus, these heroes of the movie are in a way detached from the world (time-space) around them; either it is a crowded boulevard in Hong Kong, or it is Hong Kong as a whole. Here another crucial issue arises, that of the **isolation and impersonality** of

---

[31]   With the term *being*, we mean the human subject.
[32]   Late consumerist society is the society that mainly occurred after WWII; the basic characteristic of this society is the mass consumption which outweighs mass production. The post-consumerist society is the current form of our society, broadly known as information society.
[33]   The narrative techniques do not follow any chronological order, any form of causality.
[34]   A usual montage or editing technique in Wong's movies is the reduction or increase of frames per second of the shooting.

the main heroes as inhabitants of a metropolis, starting from *Chungking Express*.

To proceed with our analysis, in order to approach the issue of isolation and impersonality of being in the late consumerist society, it would be wise to take a look at Zygmunt's Bauman terms of the **reversed synopticon** and the **outcast**. Bauman starts from Michel Foucault's theory of **panopticon**, in which the periphery is under surveillance by the center (for example, a prison where the guard is in the center watching the prisoners around). On the scale of a metropolis, a classical example for Bauman is Paris, where the central avenues and large central squares were built in such a manner after the French Revolution so that crowd control could be more easily achieved. Bauman ascertains a shift from the model of **panopticon** to the model of **synopticon**, in which the center is under surveillance by the periphery. Bauman in most cases refers to the current phenomenon of social networks where everyone in the periphery can inspect those who belong to the center. But who really belongs to the center? Those called VIPs or wealthy people in the foreground, or even mass consumers in the background. These are the three main categories of being (consumers) in the consumerist society according to Bauman. Before referring to the last category, the **outcast** or **wasted lives**, a small pause is made to describe the model of **reversed synopticon**. The model of **reversed synopticon** is linked to the fact that those belonging to the center are in a way both inspecting *and inspected by* the periphery. The last category of consumers, the **outcasts** or **wasted lives**, are those who do not have sufficient economic resources in order to consume and usually live on the borderline of impoverishment; they can be members of social minorities like homeless people, refugees, immigrants, etc.

Referring back to Wong, the main heroes of *Chungking Express* could be described as belonging somewhere between the **outcasts** and mass consumers, considering that their professional background and their lives could be characterized as **wasted**. The two main male protagonists are just police constables; the one is just called Cop 663, and the other is named He Qiwu, or nicknamed Ah Wu or just Cop 223. The three main female characters are a flight attendant without a name who breaks up with Cop 663, a waitress in a small 24-hour snack bar named Fay who starts a platonic erotic relationship with Cop 663 after his break up with the flight attendant, and a mysterious minor drug smuggler, again without a name, who is involved in an erotic relationship with Cop 223.

Their impersonality cannot be conceived of by the spectators as mere impersonality, but as **personal impersonality**. These people may have **wasted lives** if we look upon the fact that they seem lonely and desperate, having troubles with unfulfilled love affairs and living in very small apartments, without comforts and with only the basics, because of the fact that they work in posts that are not well-paid. Finally, the spectator is approaching them with seeming proximity and he is deeply moved by their everyday experiences. First, the element of subjectivity and intersubjectivity of time perception by the spectators is anything but lost. As we have mentioned above, this is achieved through the filming techniques used in *Chungking Express*; thus, we can speak about an almost paradoxical filmmaking based on time relativity, in which time relativity itself works as the means of reduction of time relativity and through its final reduction and clearing the spectator can reach this original relationship with the protagonists. If we would like to connect this relation with Bauman's theory, it is more of a **synopticon** relation, and not a **reversed synopticon** relation. The spectators belonging to the periphery are in some way clearly inspecting the center, the protagonists. We speak about an original relationship of the protagonists, brought to the spectators to connect it afterward, with the qualitative feature of the formation of Being's **identity** in the late consumerist society in contradistinction with the formation of Being's **trace** in the post-consumerist society.

Second, we would also like to mention that the purely erotic (or the deeply sentimental) element is all in all apparent in *Chungking Express*. This is given on the one hand by the method presented above that of self-reducing relativity and the isolation of the heroes. On the other hand, and on the basis of that isolation, the director uses even more slow-motion shots when he focuses on an erotic (or deeply sentimental) scene, or freeze-frame, and even more close-up scenes. The cinematography is based on making use of filters and covers that render the screen in black and white tones, or pale purple and green tones. Finally, the erotic (or deeply sentimental) scenes are musically scored with nostalgic and esoteric songs. Considering all the above, we could speak of a core set of sublime and high aesthetic values in the filmmaking of Wong.

We now move to the movie *Pulp Fiction*, by Quentin Tarantino, for a comparison with Wong's *Chungking Express*. *Pulp Fiction* shares some common characteristics with *Chungking Express*. For example, their plots may be non-linear. However, this feature of non-linearity is remarkably different to Wong's filmmaking approach of co-presence of time and sublimation. The main difference considering the perception of time in these movies is that Tarantino emphasizes not the reduction of the relativity of time and sublimation, as Wong does, but the production of more and more time relativity in real time. Thus, we could speak for a **co-presence of time** but in a qualitatively different way. To sum up, the scheme in Wong's movies works with time relativity as self-reducing relativity, while in Tarantino's movies, it works with time relativity as self-increasing relativity.

How is this achieved in Tarantino's movies? One of the most prominent characteristics of his filmmaking is the fact that it is based on the use of black humor and irony as a means of desublimation, but this kind of desublimation is qualitatively different from the perception of Herbert Marcuse's *One-Dimensional Man* (a work mainly referring to late consumerist society). Their approach could be more properly defined as real-sembling sublimation, in continuation with the notion of the real semblance introduced by Gungov.[35] (The notion of real semblance mainly refers to post-consumerist society).

Marcuse starts from Freud and his so-called sublimation. According to Freud, sublimation is the process in which the libido is brought under the control of the reality principle. When the libido is brought under this kind of control, it is delayed and transformed into an aesthetic achievement; Marcuse introduces the notion of eros to describe this relation. The artistic realm is another dimension of everydayness, so everydayness is at least two-dimensional. Marcuse argues that desublimation occurs when eros is reduced to sexuality, which results in society becoming one-dimensional, and he posits that it is unable to resist the transformations of the system of production. In the past, according to Marcuse, the artistic and literary representations of people belonging to the margins of the society, like artists and prostitutes, worked as a means of rethinking social becoming, under the scope of a possible utopia. In contemporary society (Marcuse refers to the late consumerist society), after so-called sexual liberation, these personalities are just parts of the existing social order, and thus have no serious power of negation. Desublimation in this sense is repressive.[36]

The filmmaking of Tarantino incorporates elements of classical movies, karate and horror b-movies, even cult pornography, etc., but he

[35]   Cf. Alexander Gungov, "Real Semblance Flourishing in Post-Consumerist Society," *Sofia Philosophical Review*, vol. VII, no. 2, 2013.

[36]   Herbert Marcuse, *One-Dimensional Man* (London: Routledge, 2002), 59–86.

finally manages to produce a cinema of high artistic values and acclaim.[37] To connect this fact to Marcuse, and then to Gungov, we will refer to a characteristic erotic scene of the movie. The first way that the erotic element is preserved and not lost is that the director emphasizes the use of symbols that are connected to the unconscious—interpretation/signification of the "erotic" element, if we follow Jacque Lacan's theory of psychoanalysis and what he calls **symbolic** or **symbolic order**[38]. The scene taken from *Pulp Fiction* is when Uma Thurman as Mia Wallace and John Travolta as Vincent Vega are dancing in a steak house restaurant in order to win a dancing trophy. It is not irrelevant that before the dance the two main characters are eating and the director is giving emphasis to that fact by the use of humorous provocative dialogues and by close-up shots of the dishes and the main characters devouring their food in slow motion (*oral pleasure*). Secondly, Uma Thurman (*Oedipus complex*) is dressed in men's leisure wear (*phallus*), her hair is totally black (*phallus*), and her hair is styled in a manner that gives the essence of the aggressiveness of a real *femme fatale*. This essence of aggressiveness is emphasized in the script, with the dialogue compared to "dirty talking in pornography" (*jouissance*) when Thurman demands the trophy from John Travolta (*castration complex/symbolic castration*). Then, when they dance, the camera focuses on Uma Thurman's bare feet (*petit objet a*), and John Travolta's "cowboy tie" (*phallus*) and his seductive look (*jouissance*).

The second way that the director gives this essence of eros in Marcusian terms is the fact that *Pulp Fiction* works as an infinite meta-commentary on other classical romantic movies, and also cheap karate and horror b-movies. The black humor and irony come to the fore in remarkably dramatic scenes, like the scene of Uma Thurman fainting and bleeding after a strong dose of cocaine, which reminds one of something between a classical heroine of French New Wave, for example Anna Karina, and a heroine of cheap Italian Giallo b-horror movies like Florinda Bolkan (except directed in a dramatic way), and close-up shots by

---

[37] See the list of awards and nominations of Quentin Tarantino in world-wide respected contests like the Academy Awards,the Golden Globe Awards ,the Cannes Festival, etc. http://www.imdb.com/name/nm0000233/awards?ref_=nm_awd, last accessed, January 25, 2020.

[38] Lacan's theory is based on Freud's *Totem and Taboo* and *Beyond the Pleasure Principle*, and on structural analysis, mainly as introduced by Claude Levi-Strauss. See more at: Johnston, Adrian, "Jacques Lacan", *The Stanford Encyclopedia of Philosophy* (Fall 2018 Edition), Edward N. Zalta (ed.), URL = <https://plato.stanford.edu/arch ives/fall2018/entries/lacan/>.

Alfred Hitchcock like of Vera Miles in *Psycho*. This scene is also emphatically and erotically decorated with a passionate dance by Uma Thurman (just before she falls apart) listening to a cover of Neil Diamond's "Girl You'll Be a Woman Soon", by Urge Overkill. Here we mention that even the song is not genuine, but a cover of the original love song performed by Diamond, and the singer has a deep-vibrato voice, like Diamond's. Or as Gungov puts it, following the Marxian term of converted forms:

> To cut a long story short, converted forms are a kind of real semblance, but constituting neither an oxymoron in boring everyday parlance nor a sophisticated Hegelian speculative sublation. It is semblance in relation to a genuine reality, to the social substance, to the ultimate principles of social, political, and economic life and to whatever other dimensions we could think of, but (and this is a very crucial "but") it remains real for all practical purposes. It belongs to the same genus of non-genuine appearance as many colloquial and professional expressions but possesses an unmatched specific difference.[39]

To sum up, this kind of non-linearity, as described above in Tarantino's film, works as a **reversed synopticon** relation and not as a **synopticon** relation, or—as we put it—time relativity as self-increasing relativity. The spectators are in a way inspecting the center, the heroes, but at the same time the center works as a means of **decentering** the spectator, as a **mirror** that reflects them—to refer again to Lacan Finally, however, the spectator does not meet his **imago**. The **real-sembling sublimation** does its action; here apparently the spectator is under an "original" **reversed relation** with himself and the heroes. This **real-sembling identity** is given in our analysis the term **trace.**

Let's see this transition from Being's **identity** to Being's **trace** more clearly in post-consumerist society. In order to clarify the issue of belonging toward responsibility, as it has been conceptually structured in late modernity, in relation with post-modernity or the late consumerist society that has mainly been described by Bauman, Maria Dimitrova poses a very serious question:

> The question is that both communitarians and liberals define alterity not as otherness or difference per se, but in relation to a principle (norm, majority, law, etc.) or through mutual measurement (which also implies an accepted common standard, common measurement unit even when the role of such a tool is plaid[sic] by one of the elements in the relationship in order it to be imposed as a measure upon the other). Since the others are originally excluded from the class of the same, it is very difficult to find afterward the route back to accession and inclusion in an ex-

---

[39]   Cf. Alexander Gungov, "Real Semblance Flourishing in Post-Consumerist Society".

tended area, no matter whether this is a community of representation, recognition or joint practices.[40]

The heroes of Tarantino, following Bauman, could be included in the border between mass consumers and the outcast. Like Wong's heroes, they are mainly drug addicts (Mia Wallace), or minor drug smugglers and con artists (Vincent Vega), or generally referring to the other cast characters connected with mafia affairs. What are the qualitative changes concerning their very Being? In order to reveal them, we should on the one hand consider all the analysis made above, and—on the other hand— focus again on the issue of that transition from **identity and original relationship** brought to Wong's spectators and **the real-sembling identity** (or, as we have called it, **trace**) brought to Tarantino's spectators. We have spoken of the notion of eros as conceived by Marcuse to end up at the notion of trace; we will now refer to the notion of death as conceived by Heidegger, due to the fact that Heidegger speaks about authenticity not as the ingenuity of existence but as Dasein's essential nature of existence, to end up again in trace, with the help of the two movies. Let's cite an extract from Kadir Çüçen to make Heidegger's conception clearer:

> Dasein projects a world for itself. In its projection, Dasein has always already stepped out beyond itself, and the world is not something like a subjective inner sphere, but the world belongs to Dasein's Being, which exists for the sake of its own self or in each case mine. When the factical existent Dasein chooses itself for the sake of its own self, then it exists authentically. But sometimes it can let itself be determined in its being by others, so that it exists inauthentically. Inauthentic existence does not mean an ungenuine existence. Authentic of Dasein is a modification of an inauthentic existence of Dasein, and an inauthentic existence belongs to Dasein's essential nature of existence.[41]

Tarantino's heroes seem to form an essence of **impersonal personality**, a reversed relation with Wong's **personal impersonality**. In Wong's movies the heroes originally (genuinely) fall in love (see above) and originally (genuinely) die, while in Tarantino's, they love and die **inauthentically** but **genuinely**, conceived of in our analysis as **real-semblance** or **real sembling sublimation**. We will give two examples: the first is when the minor drug smuggler in *Chungking Express* kills the

---

[40] Cf. Maria Dimitrova, "Personal Identity: From Belonging Toward Responsibility," *Sofia Philosophical Review*, vol. IV, no. 2, 2010.
[41] Cf. Kadir Çüçen, "Heidegger's Understanding of Man, Being, and World," *Sofia Philosophical Review*, vol. II, no. 1, 2008.

head of the Mafia. In Wong's films, both the killer and the person to be killed are shown in such a dramatic and uncompensated manner that the head of the mafia is experiencing what Heidegger calls authenticity *of* Dasein or death as our "ownmost" experience; he undertakes every responsibility for his actions, which lead to his death. In Tarantino's *Pulp Fiction*, Vincent Vega, for example, dies somewhere between the non-linear quick change of shots of the movie in a bathroom of a house that he has just broken into. This accidental death can in no way be characterized as authentic, but can be linked to what Heiddeger calls thrownness, Dasein's arbitrary condition in which Vincent Vega as a guard of the head of the Mafia dies on duty, conceived as a social convention, in a non-linear matrix of a **past-thrown-towards** his being, and of **his being-thrown-towards** his death. The spectator here meets the essence of the finitude of Vincent Vega. To sum up and connect it to Being's transition from the late consumerist society to the post-consumerist society, consumers in the late consumerist society are in a way **worthy**. Their consuming identity is formed under the scope of death as their ownmost possibility, thus having a primordial essence of their actions and the undertaking of their responsibilities, a full episcope (uncovered view) of the "worldtime", as Heidegger puts it. However, in the post-consumerist society their post-consuming habits are mainly linked to the fact that their **traces** are a measure of their disposability of their finitude. They focus on the present-at-hand—thus a sublated essence of death is here to get it; their essence of buying is similar to the essence of their first breath after a coma.

Considering this kind of transition, and linked to Gungov's theory, we could admit that the main heroes of *Pulp Fiction* should be characterized more as **statistical units**[42] than as mass consumers or **outcasts**. The very Being of a statistical unit, or **trace** in our care, has immediate reference to both the essence of disposability and finitude. In the late consumerist society, the spread of information, or more simply advertising as an essential component of the marketing and the distribution of the commodity, was mainly based on a **personal impersonality** relation. The consumer subject—addicted to the mass advertisements of the newspapers, magazines, and television— – was in constant pursuit of pleasure. This constant pursuit of pleasure has worked as the comparative measure of conceiving otherness. Thus, we could speak for a **differential alterity**. It is me conceiving the other consumer, probably in the large supermar-

---

[42]   Alexander Gungov, "Real Semblance Flourishing in Post-Consumerist Society".

ket or in the big mall. The supermarket or the mall, with its small separate subunits, can be described as a place producing impersonality, but the face-to-face relationship is not excluded; thus, the consumer subject was forming an original relationship with the other. The image of his self was an image on the face of the other consumer. These may be close to Levinas, but the term **differential alterity** also includes the element of the subjective time of the other consumer, and also the intersubjective time of the Other as clearly occurring from a general form of the objective time of advertising, namely the time of mass advertising. We tried to describe this relation with Wong Kar-wai's movies. The element of constant time here is nothing more than the *co-presence* of time, and the differential alterity is nothing more than personal impersonality, and finally it is nothing more than *Dasein* conceiving the worldtime authentically.

In the post-consumerist society, mass advertising has been transformed into personally targeted advertising through the collection of millions of pieces of data from the **statistical units,** the subject of the post-consumerist society. When of course we are speaking about impersonal personality, we refer to the impersonality of data collection through several internet resources and banking systems as well as taxation systems, etc. The time of the **otherness**, as time of a **trace**, can only be approached with the following example:

Imagine that you would like to go on a trip. Well, you should book a flight, accommodation, etc., and here the perplexity of finitude comes in. The seats of the airplane are finite; the number of possible flights to the destination are also finite. The number of hotels are finite, too, etc. But how will the maximum profit be achieved for each and every businessman offering the services mentioned above?

I would like to go on a trip, to buy a pair of shoes, etc. It is strange that at the start of the formation of the desire for a trip, a pair of shoes, etc. the commodity stands as itself without further determination. To be clearer, in most cases in the post-consumerist society, only a general vision of the final determined commodity exists: this pair of shoes is not in most cases the black peep-toes or the grey climbing boots, as it will be seen that there are many factors determining the final decision. We would like to say that if there is no commodity in an a priori condition to please our desire there are two options that will be analyzed. Firstly, the desire will not be satisfied; secondly, a new kind of commodity offered service will appear by the same capitalistic system of production to please us. But in both cases, an a priori insight exists, whether it is the commodity itself or the desire to obtain the commodity.

However, let's formalize a little bit. The trip, the shoes, still are not a trip to Paris or a pair of blue platform shoes. They are a trip, a pair of shoes, etc. The maximum budget that the consumer has at his/her disposition is not the determining measure. There are thousands of options to serve each and every pocket. Up to this point I do not possess but I desire to possess. This state preserves rather than encloses the open-endedness or potentiality of possessing. Should we see it more formalized, I would like to go on a trip. I go to skyscanner.com or a similar site, then booking.com, or a similar site, etc. These kinds of sites work as a huge recording surface, receiving feedback through cookies from thousands or millions of users watching that exact time in real-time, a certain destination, accommodation, etc. And...what a miracle! At the same time, a hotel room is booked, the seats on a flight are getting fewer (purchases) or more (cancellations), etc. We mention that the destination is fixed now, and we are speaking about a trip to Barcelona. The prices of the offered commodities or services in real-time (that exactly) are changing; they are making variations that could only be compared with a jazz solo improvisation. The data collected refer to the possibility of realization (a hotel room to be booked from a user of the site) but the hidden intersubjectivity between the users and the site leads to the prolonging of the limits of actualization of the desires of the user that tend to be realized or they are being realized (a room is booked, or there are two rooms left, etc.). Considering the process, although it seems intersubjective as to its core essence, it is neither subjective nor objective; the mean of the continuation is the intersubjectivity, but the mass data is an objective state, a perplexed depository of desires of millions of users in real time. This objectivity is the measure of the possibility of actualization/realization, and at the same time its subjectivity is the ratio.

The question that arises is this: is it the commodity first? Or is it the desire to obtain the commodity? Or is everything appearing at the same time in real time? The answer may be like this: the commodity that I desire...is the commodity that I have just desired...and it is also that exact commodity that I desire right now. This final scheme is the formalization of **trace** as the very being of the **statistical units** in the post-consumerist society.

Chapter 2:
Ethics, Meaning, and Sense in the Post-Consumerist Society

Introduction

In the post-consumerist society, new forms of manipulation arise. In order to glare at all these manipulating methods on the one hand, and, on the other, in order to propose an alternative, we will speculate upon the signification, which occurs from both the interaction of the statistical units[43] and those who belong to the center (those who collect and analyze the data from the statistical units). At this point, we should generalize upon those who belong to the center. Their basic feature is that they impose dominance or power upon the statistical units, aiming at manipulation or disinformation.

Following the tradition of hermeneutics and phenomenology, we will refer to Hans-Georg Gadamer and Emmanuel Levinas. The first, together with Paul Ricoeur, redefined hermeneutics as breaking with the tradition of Wilhelm Dilthey, Emilio Betti, and Eric Hirsch, proceeding to a more phenomenological view of hermeneutics. The starting point is surely Edmund Husserl and Martin Heidegger, who affected both Gadamer and Levinas. Husserl insisted on the transcendental character of the subject that seeks the truth through science, which led Gadamer to conceive of hermeneutics as the science that is based on an ontological relationship, rather than a subjective one, and linked it with a fundamentality of ethics. Levinas, on the other hand, conceived of the Other in his transcendence and with his ethics as first philosophy, moving from the ontology to the metaphysics of ethics. He claims that the relation with being is ontological, but the relation with the Other is metaphysical. Heidegger, with his philosophy, provided the notion of a being in its openness as the care for the other. For Gadamer, this openness is found in his centrality of conversation as a mode of understanding, but also following the Heiddegerian being-in-the-world, Gadamer reveals the role that history

---

[43] Alexander Gungov, "Real Semblance Flourishing in Post-Consumerist Society," *Sofia Philosophical Review*, vol. VII. 2, 2013. Gungov, following Bauman's theory of the three categories of consumers in consumerist society: VIPs, wealthy people, and mass consumers, and also the fourth category of the outcast or wasted lives, proceeds with his analysis of post-consumers as statistical units. The statistical units can be divided into at least four categories: investors, protesters, mortgage payers, and taxpayers.

and tradition play in our understanding. Levinas accused this locality of being-in-the-world (Da) as a being that is an anonymous totality that is reduced to the measure of its self-identical power.[44] And so, he is the first in continental philosophy who breaks with the I and the self, its consciousness, its experiencing and understanding, by reversing the relation from the Other to the self. The introduction is more focused on the topics of sociality: therefore, we will refer to issues like history, tradition, culture, judgment, the word, the distinction between the saying and the said, and the command.

Gadamer, moving beyond the tradition of hermeneutics in his *Truth and Method* (1975), places his two-sided critique against Betti. First, he claims that Betti had a lack of concern for method, and second, addresses his views on subjectivism. On that basis, Gadamer exposes his views on understanding not as a subjective process, but rather as ontological. Understanding is not something that the human subject—or "we"—do by reason or by our belonging to history, but rather something that happens to us. Understanding thus is not seen in Gadamer as a subjective accomplishment; it is an **event**. By the term "event", he refers to something of which a prior condition is being situated in the process of tradition.[45]

The above are strongly connected with the emphasis that Gadamer gives to historicality in relation to the nature of human understanding. There is always a past that submits us to saying **I have understood**; rather it is "we in the first place that-we understand". We should now refer to how Gadamer conceives of **prejudice**. Prejudices are integral to all understanding. He follows Heidegger here, in a more generalized and expanded view upon the understanding in a pre-given context. According to Gadamer, prejudice is based on a pre-reflective judgment, and this is polemic regarding the Enlightenment's prejudice **against prejudice**.[46] It is a questioning of the rationality that we have inherited from Descartes to the Enlightenment. Gadamer opposes the fact that the Enlightenment, with its rationalism, in a way places authority with blind obedience and domination in parallel. He points out that every person has some kind of authority, but this fact is not something based on the subjection of reason but on recognition and knowledge. In knowledge, the other is superior to oneself in his/her judgment, and this is the reason behind **why his/her judgment has priority over one's own**. This is connected with the ex-

---

[44]   An idea that is central both in Levinas's *Totality and Infinity* and in his second magnum opus *Otherwise Than Being*.
[45]   Hans-Georg Gadamer, *Truth And Method* (New York: Seabury Press, 1975), 276.
[46]   Ibid., 240.

planation that, if someone claims his/her authority, the other has to recognize him, thus to know his/her limitation, and with an act of reason itself, admit that other has a better understanding. Authority in this sense is not connected with any form of command but is, rather, based on knowledge. [47]

Gadamer's view of tradition is nothing other than how our own horizons are shifting through fusion with other horizons. He notes that "this process of fusion is continually going on, for there, old and new continually grow together to make something living of value, without either being explicitly distinguished from the other".[48] All these are grounded upon the phenomenon of understanding.

Gadamer, in his hermeneutics, rejects the **authorial intention** as the supreme criterion of textual meaning. A genuine conversation is like reading the **other person's mind**, coming to a mutual agreement with him/her on the topic of discussion. This form of conversation is based on a **fusion of horizons**; what happens in the process of interpretation is the fusion of horizon of the text with that of another reader. Therefore, the textual meaning is nothing substantial in itself, but is a form of **event**; this event is the act of reading.[49] For him there are three inseparable moments in the "hermeneutical situation": a) the understanding, b) the interpretation, and c) the application. The theory of hermeneutics is for Gadamer a science that aims for Aristotelian practical wisdom or *phronesis*, referring to how the universal can be applied to the particular and reconciliation as the common ground between hermeneutics and fundamental ethics. We will return later in more detail to this issue in comparison with Levinas.

We should focus upon the essential finitude of all understanding in this **horizontal** nature of understanding. Gadamer links it with the acknowledgment of human finitude itself. This acknowledgment leads us not to proclaim a final coincidence with the object in question (e.g., the meaning of a conversation, or the interpretation of a text), but rather to remain vastly open to new experiencing, to an expanding of our horizons. "The truth of experience has its own fulfillment not in definitive knowledge, but in that openness to experience that is encouraged by experience itself".[50]

[47]   Ibid., 249.
[48]   Ibid., 273.
[49]   Ibid., 237.
[50]   Hans-Georg Gadamer, *Truth and Method* (New York: Seabury Press, 1975), 319.

A common place of departure for both Gadamer and Levinas is Heidegger. Heidegger not only places Being within the spectrum of time, but also speaks for a Being that has a property of openness, a being for the others, as the care for Being through which an authentic potentiality-for-Being-as-a-whole occurs. Heidegger, in his *Being and Time* (1927), notes: "What has been projected is the Being of Dasein, and it is disclosed in what constitutes that Being as an authentic potentiality-for-Being-as-a-whole. That upon which the Being which has been disclosed and thus constituted has been projected is that which makes possible this constitution of Being as care."[51] But this potentiality for Being is connected with another important issue, that of finitude and Death. Heidegger conceives of death as Dasein's ownmost possibility, and this possibility is also the disclosure for Dasein's ownmost potentiality-for-being.[52] The conception of the Being-as-a-whole differentiates us from the illusory pre-given opinions of the *Das man*, which only focus on the present, and it is we with our being-towards-death that can understand our selves-as-finite and as temporal exstases between past and future.[53] Finally, we should refer to how the possibility and the power of the possible **renders possible** both our history and our interpretation of history, according to Heidegger.[54]

For Gadamer in relation to Heidegger, we could say that as far as he introduces the **fusion of horizons** and emphasizes conversation, he surely conceives a being-in-his-openness in relation with the other. Furthermore, as mentioned above regarding the issue of finitude, the finitude of our understanding in Gadamer is surpassed with the expanding of our horizons and our experience, in relation with the being-toward-death of Heidegger. The understanding as grounded upon tradition and historicality that is described by Gadamer can also be paralleled with the being-in-the-world of Heidegger and the rendering of the possible, as to our history and its interpretation. In order to deepen our analysis, we must analyze the Gadamerian **effectiveness of history** as a response to the objectivism of history. He claims that it cannot be an objective knowledge of history, but—since history is effectively at work in every process of its understanding—there should be a grounding of historiological understanding on its own history, whereby there occurs a productive possibility of any

---

[51]   Martin Heidegger, *Being and Time* (Oxford: Blackwell, 1962), 371.
[52]   Ibid., 263.
[53]   Ibid., 267–8.
[54]   Ibid., 446.

understanding that lies in truth. Effective history in a manner provides us with the intelligibility of our horizon as living beings:

> In a conversation, when we have discovered the other person's standpoint and horizon, his ideas become intelligible without our necessarily having to agree with him; so also when someone thinks historically, he comes to understand the meaning of what has been handed down without necessarily agreeing with it or seeing himself in it,[55]

Gadamer writes. Finally, a connection with Heidegger is found on the issue of the anticipatory nature of the understanding through the pre-given structures in the formalization of the pre-reflective prejudice by Gadamer.

Levinas, in opposition to Gadamer, does not find the solution to the universal and particular, of the same and the Other, in the Cartesian *cogito*; neither is it based on the Aristotelian *phronesis,* which may reduce the Other over the sameness of universality of the reason (of the state, polis-poli-tical, in which it recognizes itself as a part of the whole, based upon a general sovereignty and human solidarity). He asks whether the inhuman multiplicity, the Other (man), can signify only the logical otherness of the parts.[56] So he seeks a relationship that is prior, or primordially constituted before any unity. This relationship is sociality as the responsibility of the Other, that is, an ethical relationship. For Levinas there is nothing outside of the field of time and history; this field stands over and surpasses our epochal and temporal history of our being. The priority of ethics (as metaphysics) is extended beyond our epoch.

What is this relationship for Levinas? This relationship with otherness is established in the epiphany in the holiness of the face, in the face-to-face. **From the face-to-face,** the **thought** awakened in the face or by the face is commanded by an irreducible difference through which thought is not a thought of but a thought for. Levinas links this facing with the very mortality of the other man; thus, he breaks with the Heideggerian being-towards-death, to the death-towards-the Other. I am responsible not for my own death, which is surely a very particular moment, but also for the time of the death of the Other. That is a demand that concerns the I, but concerns me. "The death of the Other man implicates and challenges me, as if, through its indifference, the I became the accomplice to, and had to answer for, this death of the Other and not let

---

[55]   Hans-Georg Gadamer, *Truth and Method* (New York: Seabury Press, 1975), 314.
[56]   Emmanuel Levinas, *Entre Nous: On Thinking-of-the-Other,* trans. Michael B. Smith and Barbara Harshav (New York: Columbia University Press, 1998), 185.

him die alone, it is the reminder of the responsibility of the I by the face that summons it."[57] The Other is not a negative entity, but in his very positive sense awakens morality in me.

The meeting with the face of the Other is not a symmetrical relation, as in Gadamer. We are not obliged to find a common place of conversation based upon a mutual agreement; it may recognize the superiority of the other person as having a better understanding of me, but this mutuality does not permit the other to impose his authority over me. This is not something that happens, nor is it in between, in Levinas. The meeting is based on a radical asymmetry; I am always more responsible than the Other. The face of the Other, as—in a manner—the *I*, occupies the position of the Other in his fragility and nudity of the face, is the responsibility for the Other, as "the impossibility for the other man, the impossibility of leaving him alone in the mystery of death". This relation is based on love; this love is not love or eros in general, nor a reduction to altruism, the goodness of a generous nature, but it is rather an an-archic bond between the subject and the good that comes from the outside.[58] If, in a conversation, for Gadamer, the mutual agreement has nothing to do with the command, in Levinas the ultimate ethical imperative is given through the command "You shall not kill". The goodness in our Judeo-Christian tradition is something beyond being. It is the love of one's fellow man—of love without concupiscence—on which the congenital meaning of that worn-out word is based.[59]

At this point, we should speak about the language and the word, the saying and the said. Words, for Gadamer, stand at the beginning of human history and the history of humanity. Language, as Aristotle points out, is what separates us from the other animals, as humans being rational beings make use of language. Logos for Gadamer does not have the meaning of the **word**, but of the **discourse**; language is articulated in the discourse, governed by thought and reason. This brings together Heidegger, Levinas, and Gadamer, as Heidegger says that we inhabit our language and it is our home. Gadamer insists on the genuine efforts that we make with communication, what we share and make communicable

---

[57]   Ibid., 186.

[58]   Emmanuel Levinas, "Humanism and An-Archy," *Revue Internatinal de la Philoso-phie,* no. 85 (1968): 65-82.

[59]   Emmanuel Levinas, *Entre Nous: On Thinking-of-the-Other*, trans. Michael B. Smith and Barbara Harshav (New York: Columbia University Press, 1998), 186.

with others. "The word is communication, sharing in its purest form".[60] A conversation, as Aristotle puts it, should be grounded in a mutual agreement *kata syntheken*, that aims as in Greek to the *koino sympheron.*

Language is not the only symbolizing activity, according to Gadamer; he follows Ernst Cassirer's definition of culture as **the symbolic universe**. Then he claims that when we take distance from others, this belongs to such a symbolic universe to the word. By this **distancing** the word achieves two things: first the recognition of the self in another; and then recognition among the others as agreed by everyone, in our cooperation bringing forth what is just.[61]

Gadamer distinguishes three words of our tradition. First is the word of the question, as what enables us to own up to our finite contingency, and to the limitedness of our knowledge, interpretation, and foresight; in short, through it we own up to the human situation in the world. Next is the word of the legend that reveals the word's special claim to the autonomy not of the being saying, but rather to the said, as the word of the poem does. And, finally, is the word of the promise in a two-folded sense of the word of forgiveness and the word of reconciliation—the word of forgiveness as someone already is forgiven, before the forgiveness, that adopts the form of an imperative to justice. In Levinas, as written above, the highest imperative is the "you shall not kill". And finally, by the word of reconciliation, Gadamer means that it always brings an increase into the world. The otherness that divides us can be surpassed through the "reality of thinking and living in a community with solidarity, thus reconciliation is the last and first word."[62]

Levinas, on the contrary, emphasizes the asymmetry and the formation awakening of the morality of the I, not as the autonomy of the I, but as the radical heteronomy of the Other's appeal to me. The face of the Other carries importance as itself; it is always seen as exteriority, because it is not hidden behind the said, but its saying is always implicit and the encounter with the an-other takes place even in the unspoken lie.[63] Logos is for Levinas an-archic without an arche, because it questions the established order. The Logos recognizes the mystery of primary

---

[60]   Hans-Georg Gadamer, "Culture and the World," in Hans-Georg Gadamer, *Praise of Theory: Speeches and Essays*, trans. Chris Dawson (New Haven: Yale University, 1998), 7.

[61]   Ibid., 8.

[62]   Ibid., 10.

[63]   Maria Dimitrova, *Sociality and Justice, Toward Social Phenomenology* (Stuttgart: Ibidem Press, 2016), 117.

sociality. At each point of a conversation, the presence of the Other (even when he is absent), transcends every image, statement, or conclusion.[64] The face-to-face is relationship seen as closeness, and this closeness is non-intentional, and non-dimensional; it shapes all the distances that are created and defended in general; it is what Levinas finds in his *caress* and *feminine*. The feminine as the radically different permits the other subject to get in the maximal horizon of the hidden, of the mystery that can be revealed through the commonplace of caress. *Caress* cannot be accommodated through language; it is rather a relation that opens a chain of occurring multiple possibilities, of a coming to be of the mystery of the future, without content. But the alterity that Levinas describes is not at the level of "there-is", but rather at the level of the anonymous existing of being in general; thus, there is an essence of transcendence in this relation. (Here we should pause and say that this kind of relationship should not be confused with *apeiron*; the Platonic references of Levinas are just attempts to grasp this kind of Platonic **goodness** that is somehow beyond being, a kind of faceless indefinite).[65]

The above is closely related to Levinas's conception of culture. Levinas points out that culture has been made by the human in the barbarism of being. The meaning that art, poetry, and thus culture bring should be seen as the exteriority that brings this dwelling, in terms of the barbarism of transcendence and the forgiveness of the Other. Levinas points out that:

> Culture is neither a going beyond nor a neutralization of transcendence; it is in ethical responsibility and obligation towards the Other, a relation of transcendence qua transcendence. It can be called love. It is commanded by the face of the Other man, which is not a datum of experience and does not come from the world.[66]

Gadamer argues that in the contemporary world, mass production and technological achievements brought a positivistic rationality; this fact opens the inquiry upon the human being, and—according to him—man needs to be cultivated, thus to have culture. He proceeds by an analysis of the specialization and non-specialization of humans and connects it with the organ of the hand. The hand is conceived of as an intellective organ; even our intellect of the senses is inspired by the hand, as far as

---

[64]   Ibid., 117.

[65]   Emmanuel Levinas, *Time and the Other*, trans. Richard A. Cohen (Pittsburgh: Duquesne U. Press, 1987), 92-3.

[66]   Emmanuel Levinas, *Entre Nous: On thinking-of-the-Other*, trans. Michael B. Smith and Barbara Harshav (New York: Columbia University Press, 1998), 187.

we touch or feel, etc. These senses are for Gadamer cultured senses that permit us an uncontrolled prejudice, consequently providing us the capacity of choice and judgment. This cultivating is not making, but—rather—it has to do with being, in such a way as to make meaningful use of one's capabilities.[67] The hand in Levinas is connected with our responsibility to the Other, in the support of the Other in his suffering; it comes from the French *maintenir* that has at least two meanings: a) to support someone with open palm and b) holding, grasping someone with closed hand, which is connected with a) morality as carrying for the Other and b) the politics which in their power and authority need to subjugate the Other.[68] The face plays a central role in Levinas' philosophy—the face of the Other, seen as exteriority and transcendence that can go beyond being and against the totality and instrumentality of the reason of the state; even a liberal state, for Levinas, can adopt certain totalitarian characteristics, because it obliges people to become in a manner depersonalized in their following the universal laws and norms, even if the liberal state respects the differences among several social groups. The particular I is seen under the universal "we", which is the commonplace for the society's well-being and common good. Gadamer, on the other hand, calls for us to cultivate our taste—that is, a cultivation of one's capacity for judgment. This cultivation *(Bildung)* requires and enables one to see a thing in the eyes of others, and this aesthetic cultivation of a triggered sensory system leads us to have the proper reflexes when we are called to judge and therefore decide upon politics, our political representation.

Gadamerian hermeneutics as a tool for understanding the various modes of being in its political aspect takes the form of a socio-political praxis, in a liberal view. Gadamer may have a Hegelian basis here concerning the pursuit of freedom, but he views the task of freedom in history as an understanding and as self-understanding, which is something endless. Gadamer writes that "To exist historically means that knowledge of oneself can never be complete".[69] For Levinas, sociality is seen as the primordial responsibility of the Other, the response to the Other's appeal to me, and the awakening of the morality of the I through the Other.

---

[67]   Hans-Georg Gadamer, "Man and his Hand in Modern Civilization," (1980) in Hans-Georg Gadamer, *Praise of Theory: Speeches and Essays*, trans. Chris Dawson (New Haven: Yale University, 1998), 121.

[68]   Maria Dimitrova, *Sociality and Justice, Toward Social Phenomenology*, (Stuttgart: Ibidem Press, 2016), 160.

[69]   Hans-Georg Gadamer, *Truth and Method* (New York: Seabury Press, 1975), 269.

2.1 Part One: Subject to Subject Relation or Sum of Statistical Units to Sum of Statistical Units Relation

Let's imagine that we have a relation between those who belong to the center (elites) and the statistical units that are placed in the periphery. The statistical units are connected together due to their proximity; the reversed vectors connecting the periphery (statistical units with the center) are two: a) real-semblance[70] and b) trace. Let's analyze the three categories above separately. In our analysis we introduce the parameter proximity or proximal. The reason for this relation of proximity is that, if in the first place there were not this kind of proximal relation, there would not be a statistical-to-statistical unit interrelation. This proximal interrelation also has three discrete strata. The first stratum is intersubjective perception of time and space, the second stratum, intersubjective perception of desire, and the third stratum, intersubjective perception of proximity, or—better—intersubjective perception of the intersubjectivity itself. All the above strata are strongly connected with the other parameter: real-semblance; if real-semblance did not exist, then there would not be any kind of common perception between the statistical units. Real-semblance, in our concern, is the a priori condition of inter-subjectivity. The time-and-space determinateness of the statistical units is given with the property (feature) of the trace. Last but not least, we should mention that the limits of the statistical units (or the sum of statistical units) concerning time and space are between 0 and $\pm\infty$ (it approaches 0 but it is not in a purely 0 condition—Gödel's theorem—or in our concern, infinite finitude, it approaches ∞ but is also finite—cumulative transgression in our care).

2.2 Part Two: Statistical Units to Those Who Belong to the Center Relation

We should mention that there is no proximity between those who belong to the center and the statistical units. This kind of non-proximal relation is the a priori condition of the imposition of the center's power and its

---

[70]   The term is from Gungov's theory. Real-Semblances in the Post-Consumerist society are "semblances in relation to a genuine reality, to the social substance... they belong the to the same-genus of the non-genuine appearances" see: Alexander Gungov, "Real Semblance Flourishing in Post-Consumerist Society". In our analysis, the glaring (απαύγασμα) in a way helps being as a statistical unit to understand (interpretation) and resist all these (hidden) Real-Semblances.

dominance of the periphery (statistical units), or for the manipulation or disinformation of the statistical units. The two remaining interconnecting parameters are the real-semblance and the trace. The real-semblance in this kind of reversed relation works as the measure of the self-reflective intersubjectivity of the statistical-units and the trace as the mean of the connection of the periphery and the center, and at the same time is the measure of the distantiality of the center and the periphery or as the measure of non-proximity. The reversed relation of this distant (hidden) intersubjectivity is the mean of imposition of the center's dominance of the periphery. The ratio between the real-semblance and the trace is analogous to the ratio between the two intersubjectivities, that of the periphery, and that (hidden) one of the center. The revelation (not glaring: απαύγασμα) of the center's dominance over the periphery is the start not of liberation of the statistical units but the start of their mutual dependence. However, this strange analogy between the two ratios above is also the mean of any possible field (containing also the field of symbolic signification—or better in our concern, contextualization) of dominance of the elites over the periphery, due to their real-semblance.

2.3 Part Three: Meta-Analysis of Part One

When a statistical unit, let's call it Subject A, makes its opening to another statistical unit, let's call it Subject B, it tries to form an identity through the otherness, and then, after the formation of its identity, to proceed to expression/discourse with the other. For example, on a social networking site, Subject A does not meet the face of the Other so the face-to-face relationship that Levinas describes, mainly in his *Totality and Infinity*, does not exist. Subject A meets the trace of the other, which is radically different from what Levinas describes in his "Humanism and An-archy" and his "Meaning and Sense". When subject A looks at a photo of subject B, they only receive a static presence (παρουσία); this static παρουσία, in many cases, does not reflect a certain Being-in-the-world (εκκοσμίκευση), but rather is a mimetic action (πράξις μιμήσεως). This action, in many cases, is the result of the real-semblance between the intersubjectivity of other statistical units, or, even more, a real-semblance with those who belong to the center. The static face of the other is not the Levinasian *visage*, but a sublated real-sembling face that, works as an *in situ* machine of creating signs—**traces**, in our analysis. These **traces** are not the traces of the Other in the Levinasian essence for two main reasons. First, Levinas gives emphasis to the face as *visage*, in his aesthetics, mainly linking the element of personality, of the real identity, with the sense of sight, by saying that the only part of the visage that cannot lie is the eyes. He concludes that, in a manner it reflects the soul. Second, Levinas, in his *Time and the Other*,[71] tries to give an overview of the Other or the otherness in a measure of asymmetric impersonality. Based on the example of Maurice Blanchot's *Aminadab*, Levinas considers that conceiving otherness as an extreme view of reciprocity can lead to a view of the Other as an alter-ego, as someone symmetric and familiar to us, thus making the feeling of alienation almost impossible. Due to that fact, there is no real criterion of rethinking the personal stance, as the whole relation is self-reflective and gives the essence of an enclosure, as comparing someone with its alter-ego. The face of the Other cannot be seen on the face of an alter-ego, conceived reciprocally as the face of the self, but rather through such a radical heteronomy like being rich and watching your face on the image-face of someone extremely poor.

Levinas, in order to conceive human action on the level of labor and command, proceeds to his treatise of time. Consciousness, according to Levinas, is "the very impossibility of a past that would never have been present, that would be close to memory and to history. Action, freedom, beginning, present-representation—memory and history—articulate in diverse ways the ontological modality consciousness is".[72]

Connecting the above with the ethical philosophy of Levinas, we should emphasize the fact that goodness is deeply linked to what is called transcendental. Levinas, following the Bible (and other Judeo-Christian writings), approaches goodness as something beyond being. This transcendental conception should not be correlated with a form of passivity that is reduced to **eros** or a general **altruistic or generous nature**, but rather as an anarchical bond between the subject and the good that comes from outside. This kind of outside is the infinity of the Other. This time notion of infinity is also crucial for the role that ego comes to play in a general era of non-humanism (the era after WWII). The responsibility that someone has to undertake is not only in his self-regard, but also in regard to the Other. Levinas points out that "*The ego, I am a man supporting the universe, full of all things*".[73] In the process of tracing the Other, first there should be a point of reference, a third person between

---

[71]   Emmanuel Levinas, *Time and The Other* (Pittsburgh: Duquesne University Press, 1987), 83.
[72]   Emmanuel Levinas, "Humanism and An-Archy," *Revue Internatinal De La Philosophie*, no. 85 (1968): 65–82.
[73]   Ibid.

the two compared subjects that can work as a mean, as a real measure of non-reciprocity and not univocity; this process may be infinite, but rather interiorizes-encloses the above process. This is because of the tracing of the Other. The trace may refer to other common cultural or historical meanings between the compared subjects. These meanings in most cases refer to the sphere of the primordial, the eternal, and the produced signi- fiers occurring from them usually are without memory; they refer to a distant past, to beyond; thus, they do not work as means of proximity. This is the Levinasian conception of historicality. The personal element of the trace of subject to subject may be linked with the fact that a subject A and a Subject B surely do have some very personal features that dis- criminate between them, e.g., the personal style of handwriting, or the gestures of the face (*visage*). Regarding this, Levinas says:

> The other who faces me is not included in the totality of being expressed. He arises behind every assembling of being as he to whom I express what I express. I find myself again facing another. He is neither a cultural signification nor a simple giv- en. He is *sense* primordially, for he gives sense to expression itself, for it is only by him that a phenomenon as a meaning is, of itself, introduced into being.[74]

In our analysis, we talk about a proximal relation rather than an infinite relation with the Other; the metaphysical question that arises here is, how would there be differences between Subject A and Subject B? We are still following the example of a social network. As we mentioned above, Subject A and Subject B are under a mimetic action due to their real-semblance, so we could speak for an alter-ego relationship, but what is the criterion of differentiation? Is there really any visible horizon that can discriminate A from B? Concerning also the crucial fact that the subject A εικάζει περί the subject B, are we are talking about a process of μᾶλλον ὄν, since the face of the subject B is static, although subject A in its pro- cess of openness as we said in part one has an intersubjective perception of proximity or better, an intersubjective perception of the intersubjectiv- ity as itself (third stratum)? This kind of perception, as we will see after- ward, is probably the most crucial part of our analysis. In order to glare at this strange property of the statistical units, or Subject A and B, we should first make a meta-analysis of part two.

---

[74]   Emmanuel Levinas, "Meaning and Sense," *Humanisme De L'Autre Homme* (1972): 7– 63.

2.4 Part Four: Meta-Analysis of Part Two

The signs that subject A produces turn to signifiers when subject B tries to give an interpretation (ερμηνεία), and the final concept of their interrelation is the signified (the signified is in a manner a sublated signifier through the otherness). Subject A and B then stroke the center with a series of signifiers; this is realized with the property of tracing. The centrifugal direction of Subjects A and B, this direction of the **traces** contains discrete singletons *Morphai;* the real-semblance is the condition of discreteness (as it is and for the proximal relation) but they have a transitional (cumulative regression) form (they are signs that in a way are under a differential condition dx: Sign = signifier/signified). The condition that epitomizes this differential relation is given in our analysis with the term **differential alterity**. But what do we really mean by the term differential alterity? We should restate that space and local determinateness of the statistical units is given through the trace, so we could not speak about an eternal and primordial even without memory signifiers like Levinas does. The same trace in our analysis **memorizes as itself**. Or, as Heidegger says. *Dasein* is under a **constant** and **proximal** self-understating (intersubjective perception of the same intersubjectivity).

We now move to the reversed direction, to the real-semblances and **traces** that have an eccentric direction. The center encompasses the proximal again horizon of Now or Present. Jacques Derrida in his *Writing and Difference*, in his critique on phenomenology, speaks about Heidegger and his method. Derrida points out that the Heideggerian inquiry upon Being (ὄν), or being, in a way is a form of violation because of the conception of Being as Being (*Sein als Sein, Sein uberhaupt, Sein als solches)*, or because the perception of the things-as-themselves is connected with the "divine", the "primordial", the "eternal", and the "absolute" in its reduction (deconstruction). This is something that Heidegger was trying to avoid, by its vital urge to break his bond with the onto-theological tradition (Aquinas-Scotus), as well as the traditional conceptions of Being (ὄν), of the past (ancient Greek: Plato and Aristotle, and German Idealism: Kant, Hegel, etc.). Beyond this critique, Derrida recognizes one very important element in Heidegger, that he was the first who posed the ontological issue in the field/authority of the time.[75] Derrida also makes his critique of the violence of phenomenology. Derrida admits that Heidegger's phenomenological Horizon (sight) has been

---

[75]   Jacques Derrida, *Writing and Difference* (London: Routledge Classics, 1978), 90.

trapped somewhere between the maximality of the **eternal** and the proximity of **the primordial essence of the present**. For these reasons
Heidegger's seeing (ὁρᾶν), is condemned to not finding a primal start, an
ἀρχή, that could work as a real opening (διανοίγειν) to the other, to the
different, so Heideggerian phenomenology is reduced (deconstructed) to
tautologies and the inquiry upon being (mainly referring to the three
priorities of being). The only two phenomenologists who can grasp the
real element of opening (διανοίγειν) are Husserl, who speaks about the *a
priori insight*, but does not proceed to a complete theory of differentiation, and Levinas, who introduces the element of the Other and the trace
of the Other.[76]

Derrida, in his diligent theory upon the metaphysics of presence,
mainly as introduced both in his *Writing and Difference* and in his *Of
Grammatology,* introduces the notion of *differance* and *trace*. We will
briefly refer to the notion of *differance*. It is a neologism of the French
word difference; this small change in the written presence (παρουσία) of
the word in a text, although it is pronounced in the same manner, indi-
cates the change of the meaning of a word as it appears in a text, as well
as the occurring signs (παρουσίες) and of course the signification. The
small wordplay with the pronunciation is connected with the attack by
Derrida on the logocentrism of phonetics, mainly that of Ferdinand de
Saussure. Derrida admits that there is no real presence outside the process of writing.

At this point, we will give a little more emphasis to the notion of
the *trace*. Derrida, in his lecture "Freud and the Scene of Writing", speculates (deconstructing) on the memorization of the *trace*. In continuation
with the psychoanalytic findings of Freud—mainly those of the function
of the unconscious and more specifically the repulsion of trauma, and
even more specifically of the reactivation of the trauma by the memory
that Freud introduces in his *Beyond the Pleasure Principle*—Derrida
concludes that the trace concerning its memorizing character has two
main features: one is that it is relapsing, thus having a temporal character; and the other is that is repeating, and thus can power the production
of other signs and, of course, take forth a series of signification. Derrida,
based upon these two basic features, will declare the death of the writer
(the writing subject). The writer can only be conceived by the other

---

[76]   *Writing and Difference* by Derrida was first published in 1967, before *Meaning and
Sense* and *Humanism and An-archy* by Levinas, which were published in 1968 and
1972.

through its trace and make its opening with the cooperation of the *differance* and the trace; the signs that could never be presented by one writer can be supplemented by another or a writer who writes with two hands. Here Derrida pays attention to the element of the other of the reversed of the different. Later in his lecture "The Theater of Cruelty and the Closure of Representation", he will connect the process of opening (διανοίγειν) with the essence of finitude and, more precisely, the essence of Death. The trace can only make its presence through its absence; this absence is connected with the essence of temporality. Derrida ends up with this conclusion:

Because it has always already begun, representation, therefore, has no end. But one can conceive of the closure of that which is without end. Closure is the circular limit within which the repetition of difference infinitely repeats itself. That is to say, closure is its playing space. This movement is the movement of the world as play. "And for the absolute life itself is a game". This play is cruelty as the unity of necessity and chance. "It is chance that is infinite, not god" (Fragmentations). This play of life is artistic. To think the closure of representation is thus to think the cruel powers of death and play which permit presence to be born to itself, and pleasurably to consume itself through the representation in which it eludes itself in its deferral. To think the closure of representation is to think the tragic: not as the representation of fate, but as the fate of representation. Its gratuitous and baseless necessity. And it is to think why it is fatal that, in its closure, representation continues.[77]

2.5 Part Five: The Performativity of the Action and the Fallacy of Derrida

Having in mind the relation between those who belong to the center (elites) and the statistical units which are placed in the periphery, we could see (in the center) that in a manner due to the shortening of turnover times, the input of the **traces** (flows of information or dx-signs or dx-*Morphai*) is under the sovereignty of the proximal horizon of the present. Derrida connects the process of common signification with the other (διανοίγειν), with the present, with **the living present**. In the center of the center, a strange process is actualized: the overlapping of the signifiers produced by the Statistical Units or Subjects A and B. In this maximal centralization, those who belong to the center (elites, the state, eco-

---

[77]   Jacques Derrida, *Writing and Difference*, 316.

nomic institutions, etc.) are meta-analyzing the data collected from the subjects placed on the periphery, and in this vital, crucial point of maximality, a general signifier occurs that is the outcome of all the input of the information that the periphery loaded to the center. This general signifier "breaks" the continuity of time. (We can talk here about a viral video in a social network, e.g., 2000 views per minute, or the notion of the surplus value, not from the production and circulation of the commodity but the surplus value of the periphery, as Antonio Negri claims[78]; briefly we could speak for a surplus-value of the post-consumption that is connected with finitude—consumption for consumption). The fallacy of Derrida here starts to appear in the reversed relation: when the general signifier is trying to be temporarily interconnected with the periphery, the real-semblance between the center and the periphery traces the general signifier backwards. As we mentioned in Part Two, this occurs not in a proximal way, but in an inclination to manipulate and to disinform; thus, we have in reversion: General Signifier = Real-Sembling sign = sublated signified by the periphery = under a process of actualization that turns into Reality. Thus, we speak for a dynamic of attaining greater proximity. When a Subject A (the gender is indifferent) re-turns back on the re-viewing of a photo of a Subject B or—more specifically—on a fully informed profile of a Subject B in a social network, the same re-viewing functions as the repetition of a possible proximation. It is the gradual filling of the gap, the gradual annihilation of the lacking. The whole process falls back on the actual. The actualization is connected with the second part of the neologism, the -semblance. The contextualization or the possible symbolic order of Subject A, in its attempt to grasp proximity, elevates its primal position to a form of openness. This elevation is the context-to-context overlapping, and this overlapping is the topic and tropic of an actual (o)thereness. The "there is" extends forth the possibility of the "there-to-be". The "there-to-be" has its grounding, first to the re-turning, second to the re-sembling. It is more reasonable to love (or juir) with someone, and his/her/@'s actually existing order of the context-to-context proximation. The occurring homo-topics and homo-tropics, through the real-semblance, is the "self-relation-coming-to-be." But, this coming-to-be-through-(o)thereness is in sublation the re-turning to the other-to-be, or better, to actually be-like or re-sembling—to-be-like.

---

[78]   Antonio Negri, Michael Hardt, *Empire* (Cambridge: Harvard University Press, 2000), 223.

Therefore, the opening (διανοίγειν) of Derrida that may reveal the field of the dominance of the center over the periphery is not a glaring (απαύγασμα). Derrida is leading one to rethink Nietzsche through the rethinking of Bataille, and his *Erotism*. Derrida points to two basic features of writing sovereignty: (1) it is a science; (2) it relates its objects to the destruction, without reserve, of meaning. The dance of Zarathustra, or the Apollonian and Dionysian conception of dialectics, can reveal this power imposition of the center.Bataille argues in his *Erotism* that:

In a sense, the condition in which I would see would be to get out of, to emerge from the "tissue"! And doubtless I must immediately say: the condition in which I would see would be to die. At no moment would I have the chance to see! The condition in which I would see would be to get out of, to emcrgc from thc "tissue"! And doubtless I must immediately say: the condition in which I would see would be to die. At no moment would I have the chance to see.[79]

Derrida then connects this emergence of the **tissue** with the trace of the Other, but the subject is completely absent; it can only be seen as the trace of the other; where is, therefore, our Subject A and B? Where are the statistical units? Our speculative-figurative analysis could not work if we were following the deconstruction, nor this phenomenological Hegelianism: Derrida says for Hegel:

> The Hegelian *Aufhebung* is produced entirely from within discourse, from within the system or the work of signification. A determination is negated and conserved in another determination that reveals the truth of the former. From infinite indetermination one passes to infinite determination, and this transition, produced by the anxiety of the infinite, continuously links meaning up to itself. The *Aufhebung* is included within the circle of absolute knowledge, never exceeds its closure, never suspends the totality of discourse, work, meaning, law.[80]

Let's try to visualize a possible example of disinformation or manipulation of the elites. We can imagine that in the news titles, or the news feed appearing on our computer or smartphone we read that: Subject A is **violent** because he/she was involved in a series of mass killings. Just a few lines below, we read that the minister of justice declared that he condemns **any** form of **violence**, from "wherever" it comes. In the first example the action is in a manner justified; a person is characterized as violent because he/she acts in such a manner. In the second case, a per-

---

[79]   George Bataille, *Erotism: Death and Sensuality* (Los Angeles: City Lights, 1986), 222.
[80]   Jacques Derrida, *Writing and Difference* (London: Routledge Classics, 1978), 348.

son who holds authority, proceeds to an **unjustified** condemnation of violence, placing a general normative context around the possible signification that violence may have.

We see that these general signifiers directed by the elites can easily place the "correct" field of the subject's normativity and performativity. But, and this is a very important but, if we are talking about a decentered-deconstructed-saturated[81] (not non-linear) subject in postmodernity, in a way we do not speak about a real subject (the other through its trace, Levinas/Derrida, etc.); the subject (Being) is only under a certain performativity and is almost excluded; thus we could only alter the model of performativity of the subject to a performativity of the action or, better, the performativity of the action as a means of evaluation modeling. We return to Derrida in order to clarify this "almost" excluded subject:

> Turned towards the lost or impossible presence of the absent origin, this structuralist thematic of broken immediacy is, therefore, the saddened, negative, nostalgic, guilty, Rousseauistic side of the thinking of play whose other side would be the Nietzschean affirmation, that is the joyous affirmation of the play of the world and of the innocence of becoming, the affirmation of a world of signs without fault, without truth, and without origin which is offered to an active interpretation. This affirmation then determines the noncenter otherwise than as loss of the center. And it plays without security. For there is a sure play: that which is limited to the substitution of given and existing, present, pieces. In absolute chance, affirmation also surrenders itself to genetic indetermination, to the seminal adventure of the trace[82]

In conclusion, we introduce the term avulsion ($απόσχιση$) to describe the above formalizations. Avulsion ($απόσχιση$) is the phenomenon in which, into a specific representational flecnode of a horizon of becomings (events), the topological space that occurs does not create new representations, but rather produces feedback which functions in such a manner that the production of its meaning brings an a priori constant beyond every contextualization. The general indentitary signifier, as a response of the Being-into-the-horizon to Dehors, triggers a chain of signification and immanence that imposes a flow of information as unilateral feedback. The latter could have a positive, negative, or neutral intentionality and immanence.

Example: News feed/ THE FIRST LADY in the photo is among the American president, among THE FIRST LADY of Greek democracy, among the Greek President, etc. Here the imposed: FIRST LADY avuls-

---

[81]   The various theories upon the subject in post-modernity; the terms refer in sequence to Lacan, Derrida, and Deleuze and Guattari.

[82]   Jacques Derrida, *Writing and Difference*, 369.

es (αποσχίζει) Being (the person) and introduces a decontextualization of the FIRST LADY. The term substitutes the avulsive feedback (αποσχιστική ανάδραση) of the sense. The term FIRST LADY will be, in short, the infinite contextualization. It is the FIRST-LADY-CLOTHES-DINNER-OVER-COORDINATE.

2.6 Part Six: What is the Glaring (απαύγασμα)? From Aesthetics to Logic

We will refer to a masterpiece of European cinema, the film *Alphaville*,[83] by Jean-Luc Godard. We should look upon some of the main features of the movie *Alphaville*. The film starts with a glittering, of a huge projector that symbolically represents Pure Reason and is also the eye of the powerful computer A60, which controls the dystopian city of Alphaville. The first words of the narrator are borrowed from Jorge Luis Borges's essay, "Forms of a Legend": reality may sometimes be complex to transmit orally (everyday communication), but the legend (plot of the movie in its self-reflective form), incorporates it in a form, so as to be transmitted (diffuse-open-διανοιχθεί) all over the world. The citizens of this city are obliged not to ask "why" but to only say "because"; furthermore, A60 deletes the so-called prohibited words that may interrupt the well-structured being of the metropolis. They are usually words connected with feelings or words that have a poetic function in the language, such as sadness and love (lexicons without words as Derrida would say)! The protagonist of the movie is the secret agent Lemmy Caution, who comes from the outlands; when he is suspected in the middle of the movie of being dangerous to the well-structured being of the metropolis, he is interrogated by A60. We will refer to these questions and answers: 1) "What transforms the night into day?" "Poetry", and 2) "What is the meaning of death?" "To die no more". Then, when Lemmy Caution is erotically seducing Natacha Von Braun (the daughter of the professor Von Braun who created A60), he tries to transmit and activate the meaning and sense of the words, **consciousness** and **love,** to her by indicating extracts from *Capitale de la douleur* (Capital of Pain), by Paul Eluard. More specifically, when Caution is erotically approaching Natacha, we listen to her interpretation of the poem "What is Love?": "What is love? Your voice [speaking], your eyes [sight], your hands, your lips [touch—

---

83   Godard, Jean Luc. 1965. *Alphaville, Une Étrange Aventure De Lemmy Caution*. Film. France: Chaumiane.

the caress of Levinas], our silences, our words [poetic function of the silence-absence of Derrida], the light that goes, the light that returns!" The film ends with Natacha von Braun saying to Caution "I love-you"— "I love-you". The first time that Natacha says the phrase it is transmitted to Caution mechanically, with short pauses, her face (*visage*) is illuminated by the lights of the avenue; when she says each of the words, there is not any external light but the director focuses only on the light that comes from her face (*visage*); this is the **glaring** (απαύγασμα) of opening (διανοίγειν). Lemmy comes from the outlands we talking about when we refer to extraterrestrial alienation; Lemmy is a human being and so is Natacha. Natacha also comes from the outlands, as revealed to her by Caution. The final shot is the passing-by of lights of the avenue, which are placed side by side, symbolizing a coexisting glaring (συνυπάρχον απαύγασμα) or a mutual glaring. The pain and alienation is occurring from the outside (Dehors), from the pure Reason of the A60, not only from the Other, nor from the infinity of the Other, and, finally, not from the trace of the Other. Natacha falls in love with the third that Levinas describes, not the Other but the third; we have a human subject to human subject relation, with difficulties of opening (διανοίγειν) due to an exterior context, due to an absolute form of contextualization. The phrase "I love you" is the light that returns; it is the return of the consciousness and the start of co-existing (συνυπάρχειν).

The opening of the two heroes transcends not the other being, but the maxim of the signification of the center A60. The light glares on (απαυγάζει), the fleeing from the subjectivized context of Alphaville. The glaring is not any form of violence, or—as Derrida would say—a form of ontological or phenomenological violence; it acts as a salvation. But every kind of erotic relationship is usually under a fragile balance; even more fragile is an action of fleeing or escaping; we are giving emphasis to the dynamics of the relationship/action. It is a kind of "violence" of common meta-signification with the other, a common sensual "violence" of opening (διανοίγειν) to the other, or if we follow Heidegger in his *Being and Time,* temporality is the condition that makes possible the historicality as temporal substance of *Dasein's* Being-as-Being. The term historicality precedes the term history. The historicality (*Geschichtlich-keit*) concerns Dasein's ontological substance of becoming (*Geshehen*) as itself, and only due to that kind of becoming is *world history* possible. This kind of Being's inquiry is characterized by historicality. Inauthentic historicality is primordially stretched along and is covered (hidden). This is also connected with Dasein, inconstantly conceiving its "today". On the contrary, authentic historicality through its temporality (seen as the moment of vision of anticipatory repetition)—deprives the "today". Someone with inauthentically historical existence is always loaded with a legacy of a "past", and it seeks the modern. But when historicality is authentic, someone understands history as the **recurrence** of the possible; thus, a possibility will recur only if existence is open for it, fatefully. *"The existential interpretation of Dasein's historicality is constantly getting eclipsed unawares".*[84]

2.7 Part Seven: Trace and Arbitrariness in the Post-Consumerist Society

In the proximal horizon of present at hand, or the proximity of now, in the post-consumerist society any kind of desire is realized; the latter does not concern any form of moralizing but in a way glares (απαυγάζει) the vital necessity of questioning being, as well as of reconstructing the field of ethics. Ontological and moral issues arise, like 3D-printed organs that can be used for transplants[85] and sexual intercourse with robots,[86] as well as syndromes like Karoshi,[87] the use of animal proteomics as a means of producing commodities by animals of the same proteome of milk,[88] and in continuation as a criterion for identity, and through their identity of surplus value (not identity but trace in our care). Can a dairy farm product define its identity from a meticulous reduction based on its proteome? Here the term identity can be used interchangeably with the terms Origin,

[84] Martin Heidegger, *Being and Time* (Oxford: Blackwell, 1962), 444.
[85] Carl Schubert, Mark C van Langeveld, and Larry A. Donoso, "Innovations in 3D Printing: A 3D Overview from Optics to Organs," *The British Journal of Ophthalmology*, no. 98(2): 159–61.
[86] Laura Bates, "The Trouble With Sex Robots". Nytimes.Com, July 17, 2017, https://www.nytimes.com/2017/07/17/opinion/sex-robots-consent.html?mcubz=0, last accessed, January 25, 2020.
[87] K. Nishiyama, J. V. Johnson, Nishiyama K., "Karoshi – Death from Overwork: Occupational Health Consequences of Japanese Production Management, "*International Journal of Health Services: Planning, Administration, Evaluation*, no. 27 (1997): 625–41.
[88] Athanasios Anagnostopoulos K., Angeliki I. Katsafadou, Vasileios Pierros, Evangelos Kontopodis, George C. Fthenakis, George Arsenos, Spyridon Ch Karkabounas, Athina Tzora, Ioannis Skoufos, and George Th Tsangaris, "Dataset of Milk Whey Proteins of Three Indigenous Greek Sheep Breeds," *Data in Brief* 8 (September). Elsevier Inc (2016):877–80. See also: Anagnostopoulos, A. K., Katsafadou, A. I., Pierros, V., Kontopodis, E., Fthenakis, G. C., Arsenos, G. Tsangaris, G. T, "Milk of Greek sheep and goat breeds; characterization by means of proteomics," *Journal of Proteomics*, no.147 (2016):76–84.

ETHICS, MEANING, AND SENSE   63

Geographical Indication, and Traditional Specialty. There are specific criteria according to the European legislation for an agricultural or dairy farm product to be categorized as such. Do our consuming criteria in this case leave behind the geographical, historical, and anthropological traits of the product and the standardized protocols of production, composition, and processing which define its uniqueness, and end up with a consumption of a certain proteomic sequencing which stands outside a definitive context? Does the contemporary food industry and market demand such "extremes" of originality and thus redefine the relationship between local rural populations (as expressed through the products they produce) and globalism?

Is overwork leading to death connected to a lack that overdetermines the limits of our physicality? A working body starts to inscribe the variations of a possible precarity and social Darwinism, but all these social restraints from wellbeing are inversely expressed through a condition in which the subject tries to obtain pleasure and enjoyment from a gradual self-torture. Likewise, the deadline of submitting a project is equal to a jouissance.

Do 3D-printed organs and organ transplantation in general really challenge our finitude and conception as mortal beings? Do we submit to a process of bodily transformation or, from another point of view, do our bodies actively transform separately from transplantation or the use of prosthetics?

Do the redefinitions of our sexual relations, and intercourse with robots, really open up the issue of fusion of machine with an organism?

All these issues will be broadly analyzed in our chapter **Information Society and a New Form of Embodiment.**

The above issues are strongly connected with finitude, or post-consumption; they are also connected with a general persistence of eternal life in a world that is getting, on the one hand, even more liquid, and, on the other, even more violent and enclosed.

How could we escape from all this production of subjectivities, of real-semblances? Let's see it as an interplay between three parameters: a) differential alterity, b) arbitrariness, and c) topsy-turvyness. The term that we introduced in part four, **differential alterity** between the subject A and B, is the factor that "violates" the common meta-signification with the other in the post-consumerist society; it is a form of "violation" of a common opening ($\delta\iota\alpha\nu o i\gamma\varepsilon\iota\nu$). This parameter should be combined with the other parameter, arbitrariness. What is its function? It has multiple functions: 1) it reminds the other subject of their intersubjectivity like Lemmy Caution reminds Natacha of the meanings of consciousness and love; 2) through this reminding it glares (απαυγάζει) the hidden intersubjectivity between those who belong to center and those who belong to the periphery; and 3) the field of authority and anti-authority is now re-established (decontextualization).

There is also a third parameter, topsy-turvyness. Let's see how Hegel conceives it, through the analysis of Donald Phillip Verene, in his *Hegel's Recollection*. Consciousness, in attempting to grasp the object as thing and properties, has moved to a more "intellectualis" position; now we have a mere sensing of the object to a kind of thinking of it. In this procedure consciousness experiences deception because that which holds the object together as properties cannot itself be an object of perception. The new object becomes a force (*Kraft*) or a play of forces. The object is understood, not perceived. This understanding (*Verstand*) is a kind of inner force or Kraft. The understanding is a power that looks through the middle or center (*Mitte*) of the play of forces to the background. It looks to an unseen element. In this way, the opposition between the appearance and the supersensible world is produced. This twofold sense of force gives us the topsy-turvy world.

Hegel says that consciousness, in order to make itself a basis of itself, must experience the reversal of its own power of object. The deception (*Tauschung*) of consciousness now is systematic deception. It has become a trauma that shakes consciousness completely.

In the topsy-turvy world, the selfsame reality repels itself from itself and is transformed into its opposite. In the inverted world, black is white and criminals are benefactors. This is, for Hegel, not only inverted but perverted. In the topsy-turvy world, consciousness has lost its bearings. The chaos comes through the fact that the oppositions between the two supersensible worlds are equal. Consciousness has lost the function of the double sense of the *Ansich*. But, at last, itself as self-consciousness is established when *Ansich* then takes up something for itself. The directionality of opposition is now re-established.

The answer to a topsy-turvy world (*Werkehrte Welt*) is a *Wissenschaft* of consciousness that can in principle overcome the possibility that things are not in reality what they seem to the powers of understanding. Even fundamental distinctions can overcome the possibility that everything is false *(alles ist falsch)*. To overcome this possibility, a totally new sense of system which plays the self-development of consciousness is necessary, based on reason (*Vernunft*).

The route that we have been making has, in its core essence, topsy-turvyness. The two non-linear subjects under their common meta-signification have two options: either they are placed in absolute self-reference and touch their nullity (zero intentionality), or they are being reversed. The first action could be very moderately characterized as perverted. The presupposition of temporal loss of the existential hypostasis is also the presupposition of the activation of the three functions of arbitrariness and the escaping. This temporal loss is not the absence of the Other, nor the absence of the sign of the Other, in the process of the common opening (διάνοιξη). We should move backwards to Alphaville: Lemmy Caution reminds Natacha, in a face-to-face relationship, of the terms, consciousness and love, even though there are gaps of silence (nullity-zero) and intentionality from a being-in-the-world, to a topsy-turvy world, and finally to the "outlands" and the destruction of A60. Schematically, the only kind of information that can escape from a black hole is Hawking radiation, and it is we ourselves fighting (in and out) against disinformation and manipulation of any kind of black-hole field of authority. Only a speculative phenomenology can help, or better, speculative-figurative thinking in the process of morphogenetical becoming![89]

---

[89]   Paraphrase of the Hegelian "Only speculative thinking can help", though in our analysis we do not adopt *Angst* as Hegel puts it, as a fundamental characteristic of human nature.

Chapter 3:
Self-portrait in a Neuron Mirror

Of Eschatological Exteriority Introduction

In this chapter, we will first deal with so-called computational neuroscience. Computational neuroscience in general promotes the possibility of generating theories of brain function in terms of the information-processing properties of structures that make up nervous systems. This idea has its origins in the cybernetic theories of the 1940s and 50s that gave emphasis to the various ways in which information (language, signs, etc.) is shared and transmitted between humans (and animals).[90] The function of the brain is of course quite different than that of a digital computer in various aspects. The most important is that our neurons have plasticity—they grow, and evolve—and, furthermore, that the number of synapses is relatively much greater than a microchip, which is connected to a computer system. However, according to the main representatives of this theory, Patricia Churchland, Christof Koch, and Terrence J. Sejnowski. it is useful to categorize certain functions of the brain as computational because nervous systems represent the external world, the body of which they are parts, and in some cases the nervous systems themselves—for example, neurons in the parietal cortex of primates compute head coordinates on the basis of retinal coordinates. The authors continue by asserting that a physical system can be modeled as a computer when its states represent states of other systems. They propose a model of organization of the nervous system in scales[91] which are interdependent and their particular function can give us different computational schemes. There are two fundamental assumptions that are essential to the proposed model, first that sensory information is mapped in spatial maps, e.g., the image of the world in the retina, and second that most of our information about the representation of sensory information is based on their recording by single neurons.

---

[90]   Patricia Churchland, Christof Koch, and Terrence J. Sejnowski, "What is Computational Neuroscience," in *Computational Neuroscience*, ed. Eric L. Schwartz (Cambridge, Massachusetts: The MIT Press, 1988), 46–55.

[91]   Ibid., 52. a) molecules b) membranes c) synapses d) neurons e) nuclei f) circuits g) network h) layers i) map-systems.

These theoretical assumptions are considered by many as a para-digmatic shift,[92] following Pat Churchland's *Neurophilosophy* (1996), as well as new efforts by neuroscientists to explain cognitive functions, adhering to the view that *the brain represents the world by means of networks of neurons* raises serious questions. First, if we think of the mind-body problem, the brain is equated to the mind and all of our cog-nitive and experiential functions seem to stem from and be controlled only by these computational operations. Is this form of neuro-reductionism, since neuroscientists seek behavioral patterns and cogni-tive processes that can be directly explained by the activation of certain brain regions or neural structures with a certain scaling, a theory that does not account for our opening to the world towards intentionality and embodiment? The experiments on neuron mirrors that we will describe give another perspective that is closer to holism than reductionism, open-ing the field to an inter-subjective approach to neuroscience and possible relations with the theory of phenomenology which will also be analyzed in order to encapsulate aspects of our experience which cannot be possi-bly understood through this reductive approach.

Computational neuroscience was generated in late 1980s and goes in parallel with the programs of early Artificial Intelligence like GOFAI (known as connectionist). These AI programs were the first that proposed so-called neuron networks. Neuron networks are specialized algorithms with quite powerful performance and are based on a computational view of our brains. They have been used from then up to now for various pur-poses like programs of voice recognition, bioinformatics, and mapping systems.[93] The modeling and the interaction between neuroscience and computer science is given below. The cognitive functions (from neuro-computational modeling) are then modeled in computer systems by so-called "parallel distributed processing" (PDP) or "connectionist units". Emily Martin explains:

> What is a connectionist unit? It is a computer into which researchers can enter data in the form of numbers, patterns, sounds, or images. Inside the computer, there is a dense network of simple computing units, often compared to neurons. Each unit receives input signals and sends output signals over connections that have a nu-merical weight indicating their importance. Each unit "decides" the strength of its output signal by a calculation based on the strength of all the incoming signals. The units together "learn" by checking their output against correct outputs re-

92   Emily Martin, "Mind-Body Problems," *American Ethnologist* , no. 27 (2000): 569–90
93   Patricia Churchland, Christof Koch and Terrence J. Sejnowski"What is Computational Neuroscience".

searchers would provide ... As it learns, the network reweights the inputs and "grows neurons" as needed to produce the correct outcome.[94]

Emily Martin makes a two-sided critique of neuro-reductionism.[95] The first concerns the reduction of mind to body, as related to the explanatory models of psychological processes in terms of neuronal processes. She clarifies her views, following the work of Nikolas Rose, who proposes a scientific example, which is connected with biological psychiatry. Biological psychiatry conceives of the brain as a kind of thing. Depression, for example, is a brain thing. Furthermore, the brain is not approached as an undifferentiated organ, but rather as an organ which functions by the interaction of neurotransmitters on a molecular level. This conception does not much take into account the social, biographical, or environmental conditions that may have led to the manifestation of a mental illness like depression. Because it is quite easy to explain mental illness in terms of chemical malfunctioning, this led to an impact in contemporary culture mainly in the way antidepressant and antipsychotic drugs are advertised, such as simple schematic diagrams of neurons with neurotransmitters circulating between them.

The second field Emily Martin critiques is cognitive neuroscience. Her basic argument is that, since a computer performs brain tasks such as remembering and decision-making, the human brain functions in a manner similar to a computer. Consequently, all kinds of learning within culture can be reduced to networks of neurons. Furthermore, the products of history, culture, and identity now can be reduced to brain functions. In this way, "culture" is reduced to "nature".[96]

Steven Rose proposes that the problem with neuro-reductionism is that the brain is equated with the mind; furthermore, it has to do with the relation between parts and wholes.[97] It is not the brain that creates concepts or participates in knowledge acquisition, but rather people using their brains. Or to put it differently, I need my brain to think, but it is I, not my brain, which does the thinking.

---

[94]   Emily Martin, "Mind-Body Problems,".
[95]   Emily Martin, "Talking Back to Neuro-reductionism", in *Cultural bodies : ethnography and theory*, ed. Thomas Helen and Ahmed Jamilah (Malden, MA :Blackwell Pub., 2004), 190–210.
[96]   Ibid.,
[97]   Steven Rose, "The Need for a Critical Neuroscience: From Neuroideology to Neurotechnology", in *Critical Neuroscience A Handbook of the Social and Cultural Contexts of Neuroscience*, ed. Suparna Choudhury and Jan Slaby (Malden, MA: Blackwell Pub., 2012), 53–66.

Additionally, he asserts that past philosophers of mind have posed problems over qualia and first-and-third person experience, without striving towards empirical findings from neuroscience. Today, at least in the US, it seems that a relation between philosophers and neuroscientists has started without fruitful outcomes since their approaches are radically different.

Concerning the term consciousness, not from a neuroscientific view but from a broader perspective, it remains detached, for example, from Freudian consciousness, or feminist consciousness, as in the neuroscientific sense it is removed from history and culture.

Rose proposes that recent findings on mirror neurons may provide a point of view which encapsulates the fact that human consciousness is based on the interactions of biological co-evolutionary processes and culture. This view conceives of human biology as inseparable from culture and humans as biosocial creatures.[98]

Laurence J. Kirmayer and Ian Gold, against this form of reductionism, propose that the higher levels of behavior may not be solely dependent on a lower level, but also on an emerging macro level which envelops the environmental context (complex behaviors, reproduction, self-repair, and adaptation to new environments).[99]

Human behavior consists of multiple levels of interdependence and mutual interaction: the social, the psychological, and the neuropsychological. From a reductionist perspective the higher levels can be described only in terms of lower-level interaction. This is also connected with an overall biologization of psychiatry, according to which neurobiological mechanisms can explain psychopathology. The lower level of molecular biology seems to be the most prominent explanatory model of psychopathology. Of course, this assumption leaves aside interpersonal interaction and social and family environmental factors which contribute to psychopathology. The explanations are based on a neo-humoral view which approaches mental illness as an imbalance of neurotransmitters.

Thinking about "connectionist units", we reach a point where human imagination as producing *schemata* and *noemeta* is under a possible threat of nonhuman entities that imitate brain function. Although we do not speak about superintelligence, a form of AI superior to and more

98   Ibid.,
99   Laurence J. Kirmayer and Ian Gold, "Re-Socializing Psychiatry: Critical Neuroscience and the Limits of Reductionism" in *Critical Neuroscience A Handbook of the Social and Cultural Contexts of Neuroscience*, ed. Suparna Choudhury and Jan Slaby (Malden, MA: Blackwell Pub., 2012), 307–330.

capable than humans—which will be analyzed in the chapter on information society and a new form of embodiment—it seems that neuron networks can of course compute, then learn, and through this learning produce more complicated outcomes, quite similar to those of humans. If we make the hypothesis that this is a form of "imitation" of human imagination, could more advanced forms of human spirit like poesies (from general poetics up to poetry) stand as a definitive factor of distinguishing between humans and nonhuman entities? We will briefly list the main attributes of neuron mirrors, as intercalary with our analysis, that goes even further and encompasses the sphere of metaphysics, ontology, and poetics, in parallel with one of the most important poems of postmodernity, John Ashbery's "Self-Portrait in a Convex Mirror". It is practically a continuation of the former chapter, in which we theoretically exposed the process of "mutual glaring" and "mutual understanding"; this is the reason we explore the various theories of neuroscience and phenomenology that could possibly enlighten the meaning of such intersubjective understanding. Major emphasis is given to certain cases that lead to the enclosure of Being, when it attains exteriority, and therefore the opening to the world in general.

3.1 Neuron Mirrors: A Brief Overview

The studies of F5 neurons in macaque monkeys, by Rizzolati et al. (1988),[100] later identified as "neuron mirrors" by Gallese et al. (1996),[101] triggered the debate over the neuroscientific basis of social cognition and the possible of intersubjectivity. Mirror neuron activity is "a fundamental mechanism at the basis of the experiential understanding of other's actions".[102] In general this mechanism claims that since the body-brain systems of two different individuals share a common function, there is a possibility of "mirroring" or "simulation" of their respective brain areas. Gallese et al. (1996), after recording the electrical activity from 532 neurons in the area F5 in macaque monkeys, reexamined previous data which proved that the neurons in this area discharge during goal-directed

---

[100]   G. Rizzolati, L. Fadiga, V. Gallese, L. Fogassi, "Functional organization of inferior area 6 in the macaque monkey," *Experimental brain research*, no. 71 (1988): 491–507.

[101]   V. Gallese, L. Fandiga, L. Fogassi, G. Rizzolati, "Action recognition in the premotor cortex," *Brain* no. 119 (1996): 593–609.

[102]   Gallese Keysers, Rizzolatti, "A unifying view of the basis of social cognition," *Trends in cognitive sciences* 8 (2001): 396–403.

hand and mouth movements. In this area, neuron mirrors (in order to be visually triggered) require the participation of an agent and the object he uses (action-object). The actions most represented among those activating mirror neurons were grasping, manipulating, and placing. Gallese and Goldman (1998)[103] view the mirror neurons in relation with the simulation theory of mind-reading. According to them, there are some matching systems (between the minds of two agents) that can enable an organism to detect certain mental states of observed conspecifics. This could reveal a general mind-reading ability. Furthermore Gallese et al. (2004)[104] provide us with a unifying neural hypothesis on how individuals understand the actions and emotions of others. Their main assumption is the activation of a mirror neuron system. There is also a similar mechanism which involves the activation of viscero-motor centers. Gallese (2001),[105] in his "shared manifold hypothesis", proposes that the capacity for understanding others as intentional agents, beyond our mental and linguistic competence, is based on the relational nature of action. His proposition is a fusion between the findings of classical neuroscience and the phenomenological notion of empathy. Finally, Guidice Marco et al. (2009)[106] approach mirror neurons as a fundamental substrate for developmental processes, like imitation and learning—the focus on the infant's perceptual motor system in relation with Hebbian learning.

---

[103]   V. Gallese, A. Goldman, "Mirror neurons and the simulation theory of mind-reading," *Opinion*, no. 2 (1998): 493–501.

[104]   Gallese Keysers, Rizzolatti, "A unifying view of the basis of social cognition," *Trends in cognitive sciences*, no. 8 (2004): 396–403.

[105]   V. Gallese, "The shared manifold hypothesis: From mirror neurons to empathy" . In *Between ourselves: Second-person issues in the study of consciousness*", ed. Thompson, 33-50.

[106]   Marco Giudice, Manera del Valeria and Christian Keysers, "Programmed to Learn? The Ontogeny of Mirror Neurons," *Developmental Science*, no. 12 (2009): 350–63.

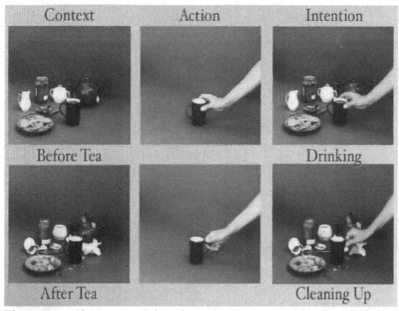

Figure 1:   Six Images Taken from the Context, Action, and Intention Clips.   The images are organized in three columns and two rows. Each column corresponds to one of the experimental conditions. From left to right: Context, Action, and Intention. In the Context condition there were two types of clips, a "before tea" context (upper row) and an "after tea" context (lower row). In the Action condition two types of grips were displayed an equal number of times, a whole-hand prehension (upper row) and a precision grip (lower row). In the Intention condition there were two types of contexts surrounding a grasping action. The "before tea" context suggested the intention of drinking (upper row), and the "after tea" context suggested the intention of cleaning (lower row). Whole-hand prehension (displayed in the upper row of the Intention column) and precision grip (displayed in the lower row of the Intention column) were presented an equal number of times in the "drinking" Intention clip and the "cleaning" intention clip. Copyright : © copyright "Grasping the intentions of others with one's own mirror neuron system", PLoS Biology, 3(3): e79, 2005, by Iacoboni, M., Molnar-Szakacs, I., Gallese, V., Buccino, G., Mazziotta, J.C., Rizzolatti, G. This is an open-access article distributed under the terms of the Creative Commons Attribution License, which permits unrestricted use, distribution, and reproduction in any medium, provided the original work is properly cited https://doi.org/10.1371/journal.pbio.0030079.g001

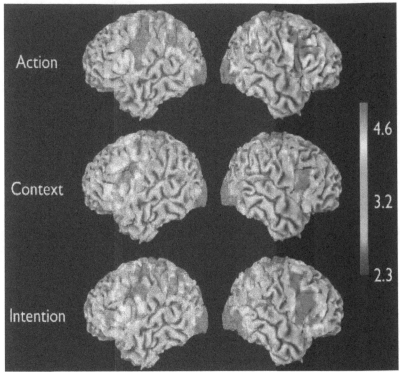

Figure 2:   Areas of Increased Signal for the Three Experimental Conditions.   Displays the brain areas showing significant signal increase, indexing increased neural activity, for action, context, and intention, compared to rest. As expected, given the complexity of the stimuli, large increases in neural activity were observed in the occipital, posterior temporal, parietal, and frontal areas (especially robust in the premotor cortex) for observation of the action and intention conditions © copyright "Grasping the intentions of others with one's own mirror neuron system", PLoS Biology, 3(3): e79, 2005, by Iacoboni, M., Molnar-Szakacs, I., Gallese, V., Buccino, G., Mazziotta, J.C., Rizzolatti, G. This is an open-access article distributed under the terms of the Creative Commons Attribution License, which permits unrestricted use, distribution, and reproduction in any medium, provided the original work is properly cited

The experiment reveals that neuron mirrors code the "why" behind an action being intentionally performed as "logically related".[107] Other surveys link the neuron mirrors as the result of strengthening sensorimotor connections that originally evolved from visuomotor control, associating the fact with the sight of the hand when we reach or grasp. Finally, the generalization is the visual observation of an agent performing an action, in order for the neuron mirror system of another agent to be triggered.[108] Is this only a mimetic action? Or is something more? Could it be, as delivered to us through critical theory (mainly that of Horkheimer and Adorno), a mimesis and simultaneously a projection, but also as Adorno points to in his *Negative Dialectics*, a contradistinction between the concept (*Begriff*) and the object (*Sache*)?: "To proceed dialectically means to think in contradictions, for the sake of the contradiction already experienced in the object [*Sache*], and against that contradiction. A contradiction in reality, [dialectics] is a contradiction against reality".[109]

In the experiment above, exploring the intentionality of the others is not only to drink or clean, as defined from extra-signified context (extra-signified as globally signified), but to set a fire. Setting a fire is to have a fundamental inclination of responding to nature, to produce not only *schemata*, but *noemata*, and this very *intellectualis* process also sublates the primal negation to contextualize, to act as opposing a predetermined series of extra-becoming as expression of an extra-being. The wood set on fire is self-preservation against cold, the craftwork of transforming a piece of wood into a means of heating.

To pass from a 1-2-3 relation to action 1 as intentionally leading to action 2 or 3, etc., is mainly linked to the dwelling among other entities, as Heidegger might say, or more profoundly the dwelling itself. To construct a table also incorporates the intention of constructing a table. Aristotle, in his conception of the universals, mentions that they exist in things and not outside of them. Arendt, in her theory of *vita activa*,

---

[107] Marco Iacoboni, Molnar-Szakacs Istvan Molnar-Szakacs, Vittorio Gallese, Giovanni Buccino, and John C. Mazziotta, "Grasping the Intentions of Others with One's Own Mirror Neuron System," In *PLoS Biology*, no.3(2004):529–35.

[108] Cecilia Heyes, "Tinbergen on Mirror Neurons," *Philosophical Transactions of the Royal Society of London. Series B, Biological Sciences*, no. 369 (2014) See also : Giudice, Marco Del, Valeria Manera, and Christian Keysers. "Programmed to Learn? The Ontogeny of Mirror Neurons," *Developmental Science*, no12 (2009): 350–63 See also: Antonio Casile, Vittorio Caggiano, and Pier Francesco Ferrari "The Mirror Neuron System: A Fresh View," *The Neuroscientist : A Review Journal Bringing Neurobiology, Neurology and Psychiatry*, no.17 (2011): 524–38.

[109] Theodor Adorno, *Negative Dialectics* (New York: Seabury Press, 1973), 144–45.

claims that it is spent in the things produced by human activity. Further-more, men constantly create their own, self-made conditions, through which the human origin and its variations hold the conditioning power as in natural things. Thus, we have a relation in which human life immedi-ately connects to a character of a condition of its existence, namely the *Human Condition*.[110]

And here is our crucial step of (o)thereness. Even in a purely sub-jectified context where being conceives appearances (flows of infor-mation) as purely transitional singletons, there is a(n) (o)therness which links, on the one hand, and on the other, permits an insight of reflection (if we could not say reflection itself), as in the walk of the schizoid of Gilles Deleuze that returns to the very same result.[111] Schizophrenia[112] and autism[113] are spectrum disorders and are linked to the fact that in the former we cannot grasp reality, while in the latter we cannot grasp the intentions of the others. And in John Ashbery' "Self-Portrait in a Convex Mirror", we have:

> A breeze like the turning of a page
> Brings back your face: the moment
> Takes such a big bite out of the haze
> of pleasant intuition it comes after.
> The locking into place is "death itself".

3.2 The Critique of Mirror Neurons by Gregory Hickok

Gregory Hickok places his critique against mirror neurons in eight points:[114]

1. There is no evidence in monkeys that mirror neurons support understanding

---

[110] Hannah Arendt, *The Human Condition* (Chicago: The University of Chicago Press, 1988), 9.

[111] Gilles Deleuze and Félix Guattari, *Anti-Oedipus: Capitalism and Schizophrenia*, trans. Robert Hurley, preface Michel Foucault, introduction Mark Seem (Minneapolis: University of Minnesota Press, 1984), 35.

[112] R. Tandon, W. Gaebel, R. Barch, M. Bustillo, J. Gur, R. E. Heckers, S. Carpenter, W. Definition and description of schizophrenia in the DSM-5. *Schizophrenia Research*, (October, 2013).

[113] McPartland, James C., Brian Reichow, and Fred R. Volkmar "New Research: Sensi-tivity and Specificity of Proposed DSM-5 Diagnostic Criteria for Autism Spectrum Disorder," *Journal of the American Academy of Child & Adolescent Psychiatry, no.*51 (2012): 368–83.

[114] Gregory Hickok, "Eight Problems for the Mirror Neuron Theory of Action Under-standing in Monkeys and Humans,"*J Cogn Neurosci* 21, no.7 (July 2009): 1229–43.

According to mirror neuron theory, if a disruption is made in F5 motor areas, there will be deficits in action perception. Although disruption seems to affect grasping behavior, action perception seems to be unaffected.[115] Hickok presents three experiments to support this claim. The first[116] regards the fact that some mirror neurons (15%) respond to action-associated sounds presented in isolation (cracking peanut shells, ripping paper). If mirror neurons are associated with understanding action, they should reflect the meaning of the observed action, not its visual features. Hickok argues that this experiment reveals that there is a form of simple association in these cases. The animal associates the action of breaking the peanut and, when hearing only the sound, activation spreads to F5, with no reflection of a meaning.

The second experiment is related to the fact that mirror neurons do not respond to pantomimed actions, but they respond only when the action is directed towards an object which is hidden behind a screen but the monkey knows of its existence.[117] Hickok, providing relevant research, claims that the monkey represents the object in working memory with the same systems that represent the object when present.

The third experiment is connected with the mirror neurons found in the inferior parietal lobule.[118] In this case monkeys were trained in grasping-to-eat and grasping-to-place actions. Fogassi et al. conclude that the monkey did not only recognize the goal of the observed motor act, but also was capable of discriminating the motor act as being part of a chain leading to the final goal of the action, thus revealing the intention of the act. Hickok again argues that this is a case of associating sensory events with a particular motor act and not because the monkey can really read the intention of the act.

2.   Action understanding can be achieved via non-mirror neuron mechanisms

---

[115]   L. Fogassi , Gallese V., Buccino G., Craighero L., Fadiga L., Rizzolatti G., "Cortical mechanism for the visual guidance of hand grasping movements in the monkey: A reversible inactivation study", *Brain* 124, no.3 (2001): 571–86.

[116]   E.Kohler, Keysers C., Umilta MA., Fogassi L., Gallese V., Rizzolatti G., "Hearing Sounds, understanding actions: action representation in mirror neurons," *Science* 297, no.5582 (2002): 846–48.

[117]   M.Umilta, Koheler E., Gallese V, Fogassi L., Fadiga L., KeysersC., Rizzolatti G., "I know what you are doing. A neurophysiological study," *Neuron* 31, (2001): 155–65.

[118]   L.Fogassi, Ferrari PF., Gesierich B., Rozzi S., Chersi F., Rizzolatti G., "Parietal lobe:from action organization to intention understanding," *Science* 308, no. 5722 (2005):622–67.

Hickok refers to a neural network beyond F5 cells that can be a candidate for action understanding. The meaning of the action can be processed in this region and then with associative mechanisms access F5 cells to trigger motor actions. This alternative area to mirror neurons could be the superior temporal sulcus. This area in macaque monkeys is connected with a wide range of actions such as reading, retrieving, manipulating, and picking. These cells, although they do not have motor properties, do not fire during action execution; they are involved with providing output to the area F5.[119]

3. M1 contains mirror neurons

The possible existence of homologues of mirror neurons in humans was investigated by indirect methods such as PET, fMRI, EEG, and TMS, which measure activity in very large populations of neurons. The existence of mirror neurons in the M1 region, which is connected with low-level motor circuiting, may generate the hypothesis that mirror responses are nothing more than the facilitation of the motor system through learned associations.[120]

4. The relation between macaque mirror neurons and the mirror system in humans is either non-parallel or undetermined

Hickock promotes the idea that mirror neurons are generalized to humans without systematic validation. A TMS experimental study of humans, stimulating the primary motor cortex to activate motor control potentials in hand muscles, has two main findings. First, concerning actions, a mirror system should exist in humans for associating observed actions. Second, concerning objects, since viewing objects does not trigger motor facilitation, humans do not have a "canonical neuron" system like monkeys and should not be able to grasp objects. Something that in any case is right, because humans can for sure grasp objects.[121]

In another study, that of Rizzolatti et al. 1996,[122] to which Hickock refers, human participants examined for grasping actions showed that

---

[119] Gregory Hickok, "Eight Problems for the Mirror Neuron Theory of Action Understanding in Monkeys and Humans".

[120] Gregory Hickok, *The Myth of Mirror Neurons: The Real Neuroscience of Communication and Cognition* (W. W. Norton & Company, 2014), 68–98.

[121] Ibid.,78.

[122] G. Rizzolatti, Fadiga L., Matteli M., Bettinardi V., Paulesu E., Perani D., Fazio F., "Localization of grasp representations in humans by PET: 1. Observation versus execution," *Exp Brain Res* 111, no.2 (1996): 246–252.

Broca's area, which is considered the human homologue to the monkey F5 area, responded during observation, but did not respond during execution or grasping actions. Instead, other parts of the brain were activated, like the primary motor cortex, the adjacent somatosensory cortex, etc. This could be evidence against the existence of a human mirror system. Furthermore, Broca's area consists of two major areas: a posterior portion called the pars opercularis, and an anterior called the pars triangularis. In the experiments of Rizzolatti et al., the human part activated was pars triangularis during object observation, but the part which activated in monkeys is the pars opercularis, so the experiment was not able to detect an activation of a part of the Broca's area during observation and execution, but only during observation, and the part detected was not in the right spot.

Additionally, Hickok proposes that recent studies like those of Rizzolatti and Craighero (2004),[123] exploring the activation of mirror neurons during the perception and execution of meaningless moments in humans, move the debate from a conception of mirror neurons as a mechanism of action understanding to a mechanism of imitation, something remarkably different, since monkeys do not imitate. This could possibly be related to more advanced evolutionary processes developed in humans that support imitation learning.

5. Action understanding in humans dissociates from neurophysiological indices of the human mirror system.

Hickok refers to a study of Brucino et al. (2004),[124] which examines the perception of actions performed by a human lip-reading, a monkey lip-smacking, and a dog barking. The activation of mirror neuron regions happened only during the performing of lip-reading by humans and lip-smacking by monkeys but not during the dog barking. If we suppose that all the participants understood the actions, this means that action understanding can happen without the intermediation of a mirror system. Additionally, Hickok emphasizes the fact that people can understand actions that they have never produced, like the sound of the saxophone even if they are not able to play it, or—in another case—an object-directed ac-

[123] G. Rizzolatti, Craighero L., "The mirror-neuron system," *Annu Rev Neurosci* 27, (2004): 169–92.
[124] G. Buccino, Lui F., Canessa N., Patteri I., Lagravinese G., Benuzzi F., Porro CA., Rizzolatti G., "Neural circuits involved in the recognition of actions performed by nonconspecifics : an FMRI study," *J Cogn Neurosci* 16, no. 1 (2004): 114–126.

tion (throwing a ball) which would result in the very same action, while an opposite action is required like catching or blocking.

6.   Action understanding and action production dissociate

We lack evidence that deactivation of the monkey mirror system can disrupt action understanding. Considering the human mirror system, there should be a correlation between action understanding and action production. Hickok, by providing specific research studies to the field, mainly in cases of apraxic patients and patients with focal brain lesions, reveals that action production and understanding strongly dissociate.

7.   Damage to the inferior frontal gyrus is not connected with action understanding deficits

Although mirror neuron theorists hold the view that action concepts involve a mirror neuron system, there is evidence that temporal lobes could be the location of action concept knowledge. Findings from a survey of patients with primary progressive aphasia support association between gesture recognition deficits related to degeneration of the superior temporal gyrus, not the Broca's area. Another links damage to the posterior middle gyrus and the ability to recognize the meaning of manual gestures like hammering.[125]

8.   Generalization of the mirror system to speech recognition fails on empirical grounds

Damages to the Broca's area should result in action understanding deficits. More specifically, patients with Broca's aphasia should have speech recognition problems that parallel their speech production deficits, yet they do not. Those people have good auditory comprehension of speech. In the case the mirror neuron theory of action was right, Broca's aphasia should not exist.[126]

3.3 Phenomenological and Hermaneutical Overview

The key solution can be found in phenomenology. First concerning Kant, Edmund Husserl extends the field of perception, as the *a priori insight.*

---

[125]   Gregory Hickok, *The Myth of Mirror Neurons: The Real Neuroscience of Communication and Cognition,* 415.
[126]   Gregory Hickok, "Eight Problems for the Mirror Neuron Theory of Action Understanding in Monkeys and Humans,".

For Husserl, both ego and world can be conceived as *noemata* through transcendental inquiry. Our capacity to be transcendental subjects functions as being able to achieve a reflective distance from our own natural way of being in the world and therefore to understand the "way" of being in a more profound way. In his *Cartesian Mediations* (1931), he introduces the conception of intersubjectivity as "reduction to the sphere of ownness". The production of meaning by subjectivity is actually cut off from others and the world and thus phenomenology is a reconstruction and not a creation of meaning. For Husserl any grasp of others as objects takes as its essential characteristic the appreciation of them as experiential subjects. In his transcendental theory of empathy, we meet his "reduction to the sphere of ownness" which is a discarding of all the experiential structures that incorporate or presuppose a sense of the others, what is world from "all constitutional effects of intentionality relating immediately or mediately to other subjectivity". In his *Lectures of Phenomenology of Inner-Time Consciousness* (1928), he makes some critical distinctions: first, between transcendental temporal objects and, second, as to our perception of them. He claims that our perception of a temporal object can be taken as a temporal object itself. Therefore, we situate our transcendental happenings in the context of objective time, and we also situate our perception of them in the horizon of immanent time. In order to clarify the conception of Horizon by Husserl, we cite an extract from his *Ideas*:

> What is now perceived, and what is more or less clearly co-present and determinate (or at least somewhat determinate), are penetrated and surrounded by an obscurely intended to horizon of indeterminate actuality. ... [An] empty mist of indeterminacy is populated with intuited possibilities or likelihoods, and only the "form" of the world, precisely as "the world" is predelineated. Moreover my indeterminate surroundings are infinite, the misty and never fully determinable is necessarily there. ... This horizon, however, is the correlate of the components of undeterminateness essentially attached to experiences of physical things themselves; and those components—again, essentially—leave open possibilities of fulfillment, which are by no means completely undetermined, but are, on the contrary, motivated possibilities *predelineated with respect to their essential type*.[127]

Max Scheler admits that our perceptual experience of others as animate organisms is pre-theoretical. He focuses on cases in which we may express fellow feelings or pity to someone and claims that empathetic and sympathetic experiences of this nature presuppose a basic apprehension

---

[127]   Edmund Husserl, *Ideas Pertaining to a Pure Phenomenology and to a Phenomenological Philosophy*, trans. Kersten, F. (The Hague: Springer Netherlands, 1982), 52.

of others as experiential subjects. The other is already given as "one like me", beyond any transference of feeling between self and other. He is not an internal consciousness that shapes a perceivable body; the other is a topos of experience. Experience presents itself in the visible expressions of the other and is grasped as immediacy. It is in the blush that we perceive the shame, in the laughter joy, etc. This is the "primitive givenness" of the others.[128]

Merleau-Ponty, in his theory of intersubjectivity, mainly in his *Visible and Invisible*, introduces the so-called *chiasm*. The chiasm is a solution to the three Husserlian types of Horizons—internal, external, and temporal. That is the interweaving between the various aspects of being and among the perceived and the perceiver, and also the visible and visible. It is the becoming others and simultaneously becoming the world. The locus of the language as the *most valuable witness to Being* can be connected with Lacan as the articulation before the letter, as deeply rooted in experience.[129] Merleau-Ponty also accounts that the others are encountered perceptually. My own body is a sense-giving orientation, through which all experience is structured. He bases his intersubjective understanding in the way infants relate with others. The response of young infants to facial expressions and their ability to imitate them do not relate to inference or analogy; infants do not have the developed perceptual appreciation of their bodies required to map the others' actions on their own, so there should be a direct mapping between perception and proprioception. He says that if we are a consciousness that turns towards things, we meet in things the actions of the others and find a meaning in them, as far as they indicate possible activities of our bodies. Both Scheler and Merleau-Ponty acknowledge that, in intersubjectivity, the self and the other emerge as separate beings; this is something that mirror neurons can indicate (ways of perception and action).[130]

Gadamer, in his *Enigma of Health*,[131] poses the question as to whether self-consciousness is equal to a theoretical objectification, which could also be similar to the objectification acquired by an artifact or a tool. He expands his thoughts on cybernetics and automation technolo-

[128]   Matthew Ratcliffe, "Phenomenology, Neuroscience, and Intersubjectivity," in *A Companion to Phenomenology and Existentialism,* ed. Hubert Dreyfus and Mark A.Wrathall (London:Blackwell, 2006), 329–345.
[129]   Bernard Cullen, "Philosophy of existence 3, Merleau-Ponty", in *Twentieth-Century Continental Philosophy*, ed. Richard Kearney (London: Routledge, 1994), 86–107.
[130]   Matthew Ratcliffe, "Phenomenology, Neuroscience, and Intersubjectivity".
[131]   Hans-Georg Gadamer, The Enigma of health The Art of Healing in a Scientific Age, trans. Jason Gaiger and Nicolas Walker (Cambridge: Polity Press, 1996), 18–36.

gies, asking if they could substitute for human labor on the level of practical know-how and if this kind of automation can affect social practice and therefore further dissolve the boundaries between human and machine. In order to propose a basis far from this fusion of human and machine, he makes a distinction between practice and knowledge. He ends up concluding that knowledge also refers to medical praxis because knowledge can be transmitted without action, without practical know-how. Furthermore, he makes a second distinction between our capacity for judgment over knowledge so as to illuminate the fact of the over-abundance of information on practical knowledge and science.

Modern medical praxis in its direct relation with theory can be exemplified today when a doctor uses such a specialized technology that permits the doctor to expose the patient to the anonymity of clinical apparatus. Practical technologies lead the doctor to judge based on appearances and thus reduce the distance between a general scientific knowledge and the current decisions of the moment. This also opens the critical issue of the *medical authority* of the doctor as the one *who knows*, something that makes us conceive an intensified illusion of the *rational forms* of decision-making. From another point of view, the horizon of the specialist becomes focused on the methodological and intellectual state of specialty.

Furthermore, Gadamer poses the issue of the capability of machines to properly exhibit the neurophysiological state of memory (*mneme*); they can also imitate recollection or at least passive recollection. In any case, the machine does not have know-how because forgetting and finding out is not know-how.

Finally, he ends up by saying that simple know-how, as specialization, in any case, is connected with the higher dimension of the spiritual domain known in German as *Gesitwisseenschaften* or as *letters* in French, or simply humanities, which also encompasses economy, law, language, and religion.

In another passage, Gadamer refers to Kant's *Critique of Judgment* and the conception of a living thing as a unified organism.[132] Gadamer follows with Hegel, who claims that life is something like the *universal blood*. This is not like the circulation of the blood, but more an organic unity of the higher animals. For Hegel, consciousness must be grasped as the unity of simplicity and finitude. Gadamer states

---

[132]   Ibid., 144.

Consciousness must be grasped as the unity of simplicity and infinitude. We recognize immediately that infinitude is constitutive of consciousness. We are always capable of thinking beyond things, and the reflexive structure of self-consciousness is characteried precisely by the capacity to progress through unlimited stages of reflection. It is this which constitutes self-consciousness as reflexivity. But alongside this infinite or unlimited character, consciousness is, at the same time, unity and simplicity. That which is in consciousness is not simply sustained in the universal blood like everything else, but is rather unified in such a way that it becomes something singular for me. Here I would like to use Hegel's famous expression, 'being for itself'. By this Hegel meant that what I am aware of is at the same time something which belongs to me. It is 'for' me. I am the one who has seen it. With this a very great step is taken, the step towards language by means of which everythingbecomes something intended by me. Whatever I can become conscious of I make my own through the speaking and using of words. This is not theplace to show how Hegel presents the transition from the stage of individualconsciousness to that of 'objective spirit' or how, as a form of spirit which has become objective to us, objective spirit is no longer to be conceived of simply as the abstract thought of universality. [133]

3.4 On Speculative Poetics

Poetry not only questions the "there is" (Da), but extends forth the ontological Priority of Being. Speculation, like John Ashbery's "Self-Portrait in a Convex Mirror", means questioning the same "poesies" and therefore the same "imaginative intentionality and spiritual intuition".

> Its hollow perfectly: Its room, our moment of attention.
> That is the tune but there are no words.
> The words are only speculation.
> (From the Latin *speculum*, mirror):
> They seek and cannot find the meaning of the music.

Poesies in a speculative phenomenological perception is the "glaring" of the very fundamental modes of Being. The very "Am I? What is there? How it could be if?" is similar to the passing from the other side of self-relation to the enchanting phenomenon of expression, the passing by of the mirror. As Gilles Deleuze posits:

> To pass to the other side of mirror is to pass from the relation of denotation to the relation of expression—without pausing at the intermediaries, namely, at manifestation and signification. It is to reach a region where language no longer has any relation to that which it denotes, but only to that which it expresses, that is, to

---

[133]   Ibid., 144.

sense. This is the final displacement of the duality: it has now moved inside the proposition.[134]

In figures 1 and 2 of the Appendix, we see the main atriums of Guggenheim New York and Guggenheim Bilbao. The selection of the two twin museums is not random. The first, as to its meta-narratives, is built in New York, symbolizing the maxim of industrialization of American post-industrial capitalism. The main exhibits cover the modern and early postmodern era. The second represents the autonomy and the seeking of identity of Bilbao; its permanent exhibition covers the spectrum of postmodern art. The two atriums form a feeling of clinamen; the conceptual diagram figure (3) depicts the transition of signification between the historicality as a context of Global Signification and the internal signification of the Being. It is an attempt at a formalization of Dehors from the narratives of the late consumerist society to the post-consumerist society. The method follows Lacanian psychoanalysis and incorporates elements of speculative phenomenology to "glare" the passing to a more nomadic and schizoanalytic approach. As Gilles Deleuze points out:

> On the very lowest level of interpretation, this means that the real object that desire lacks is related to an extrinsic natural or social production, whereas desire intrinsically produces an imaginary object that functions as a double of reality, as though there were a "dreamed-of object behind every real object," or a mental production THE DESIRING-MACHINES as behind all real productions.[135]

In figure 3 of the Appendix is presented the input and the lacking output of the Global-General Signifiers as well as the production of the S-Signifiers, (The Global-General Signifiers as the contextualization of performativity and immanence occur from the narration of the same place and the exhibits, defining a Dehors). The point of the Chiasme is simultaneously a line of non-fleeing and of production of S-Signifiers (Temporal Superimposition). The relation above forms a paradox of both positive and negative information entropy. The points of intercept are the intercepts of the architectural and artistic narrations and, in parallel, the points of the Chiasme. The events occur in a sublated way. The possibility gives its place to actuality and the real-sembling reality[136] to reality.

---

[134]   Gilles Deleuze, *Logic of Sense*, Trans. Constantin V. Boundas (London: The Athlone Press, 1990), 15.

[135]   Gilles Deleuze and Félix Guattari, *Anti-Oedipus: Capitalism and Schizophrenia*, trans. Robert Hurley, preface Michel Foucault, introduction Mark Seem (Minneapolis: University of Minnesota Press, 1984), 25–26

[136]   Alexander Gungov, "Real Semblance Flourishing in Post-Consumerist Society, *Sofia Philosophical Review*, vol. VII, No. 2, 2013. Real-semblaces in the post-consumerist

In the center we have the mirror-reflections both of reality and the real-sembling reality. The eventual time of the horizon is always interwoven with the time of producing real-semblaces and is objectified or subjectified in relevance with the objectification or the subjectification of the Being. The ratio between the objectification and the subjectification is analogous to the ratio of positive reality/real-semblance and negative reality/real-semblance. Thus we have: Possibility = Actuality (1), symbolic = real-sembling (2), subjectification/objectification = (+reality/real-semblance)/(-reality/real semblance). The non-becoming and non-eventual time of the horizon is connected with the passive synthesis or better neutrality. It occurs when the assemblages of the positive information entropy of the periphery are equal to the negative; thus, the information entropy of the periphery turns into zero condition. The being seems to be in between but always has the property of (o)thereness, so it can have an insight into the process.

Freedom is conceived as ontical, and the Being as in itself. Then the Being for itself is a being that co-transcends through (o)thereness, finally the Being in itself—for itself is conceived as ontico-transcendental. This scheme is not a play of *Vorstellung* and *Darstellung*. The gap of information flow or the blockage of information over-flow is not the voids of Lacan. It is the sharing of a mutual understanding of everydayness; simultaneously the "Mitte" of the possible self-relation is surpassed through the common meta-signification of the dwelling with the otherness as formalized "Dehors". The "mitte" is always "there" (Da). The "glaring" is like at the end of John Ashbery's poem:

> A convention. And we have really
> No time for these, except to use them
> For Kindling. The sooner they are burnt up
> The better for the roles we have to play.
> Therefore I beseech you, withdraw that hand,
> Offer it no longer as shield or greeting,
> The shield of a greeting. Francesco:
> There is room for one bullet in the chamber

This image (*Bild*) is like the Socratic: Those who rightly philosophize are practicing to die (οἱ ὀρθῶς φιλοσοφοῦντες ἀποθνῄσκειν μελετῶσι).[137]

---

society are "semblances in relation to a genuine reality, to the social substance ... they belong the to the same-genus of the non-genuine appearances."

[137] See: Donald Phillip Verene, *Speculative Philosophy* (Lanham, Maryland: Lexicom Books, 2009), 13.

The Being is finite and towards its nullity (zero intentionality) and at the same time dwelling towards "Dehors".

Jacques Lacan, in his fifth seminar, introduces his analysis of the *sign*, *signifier* and the *trace*.[138] We stop here to compare them with

---

[138] Over the last years it seems that many efforts have been made to bridge classical psychoanalysis and neuroscience. Of course, there is a serious methodological gap between them, if we consider that Freud mainly and his successors put more emphasis on psychological predispositions of psychodynamic processes. The newly-established field of neuropsychoanalysis has its origins in the first era of Freud, working as a neurobiologist and more particularly, his manuscript "Project of a Scientific Psychology" (1895). In our analysis, we will focus mainly on the work of Carolina Escobar, Francois Ansermet and Pierre J. Magistretti, in their paper "A Historical Review of Diachrony and Semantic Dimensions of Trace in Neurosciences and Lacanian Psycoanalysis" (Escobar c, Ansermet F and Magistreti PJ, "A Historical Review of Diachrony and Sematic Dimensions of Trace in Neurosciences and Lacanian Psycoanalysis," *Font.Psychol*, no.8 (2017): 734.), in order to encompass a more materialistic view, in our general treatise on the notion of the **trace**. According to the authors, the term trace historically comes from Plotinus, as the description of a passive condition produced by events, and later on by Pierre Nicole (1632–1704), who gives a theological approach of a tabula rasa, in which the sensory experiences leave a trace in the mind. To cut a long story short, they explore and distinguish the terms introduced by Freud such as: *mnesic trace* (which is used today interchangeably with the term *enrgram* and refers to cerebral plasticity and memory consolidation), *deferred action*, *hallucination*, in comparison with the "Cybernetic theory of the trace with the modal model", that of consolidation, learning, and long-term memory, "the multiple traces theory and reconsolidation", and, finally, "top down" models and phenomenology. Very grossly, if we follow Freudian thought, memory belongs to the sphere of the unconscious and we become conscious only of very a small percentage of our memories, which consist of traces. If we stick to the first associationist accounts of Freud, the various memorial strata are continuously rearranged and our percepts can be linked together with a simultaneous presentation. This scheme becomes more complicated during the activation of a trauma both from a psychoanalytic point of view and – more importantly to our analysis – from a biological point of view. In a state of urgency (trauma) a neuronal excitation is observed; the subject is submitted to the so-called pleasure principle. During this state, it tries to retain, or to obtain satisfaction in order to avoid displeasure. This avoiding is facilitated by neuronal pathways, related to the subject's past experiences, which can reduce the excitation. The facilitation maintains a *hallucinatory* character, as interplay between the reality and the pleasure principle. *Deferred action*, lastly, refers to the two phases of the traumatism; in the first phase there is no inscription; in the second phase, a second scene can impose a signification onto a past experience in which there was no association with traces inscribed before. We will refer to Hebb (1949) and his idea of "neuronal assembly", in which the trace is presented as the increase of connective strength between populations of interconnected neurons and parallel cell co-activation. According to the positivist accounts of the '40s, the term *memory* is replaced by the term *learning*; the cybernetic theory of that age was appealing more to the way information is transmitted between humans (and animals). Atkinson and Shiffrin proposed the "modal model"; in this model we find terms such as: *sensory memory (SM)*, *short-term memory (STM)*, and *long-term memory (LTM)*; the last, seen as autobiographical memory, is closer to the *trace*. In 1997, Nadel and Moscovitch delivered us the "Multiple Trace Theory"; they highlight the episodic character of memory trace is placed in the linked ensembles of the hippocampal complex; the existence of trace depends on semantic assemblies at the time of trace reactivation. In recent years we have the emergence and broadening of the model just described above, of the so called "Reconsolidation Hypothesis" which suggests the malleability of the

Jacques Derrida. Both Derrida and Lacan speak in their theories of lacking. Lacan, as reconstructing Claude Levi-Strauss's theory on canonical form, will later introduce the Schema-I and the neologisms of *lalangue* and *plein forme* (complete form), in his attempt to grasp the whole of the chains of unconscious. The lacking in Derrida is formalized through its *trace* and *differance*, as well as his dangerous supplement. But where do these series of signification stop?

Lacan, in his twentieth seminar of the Encore, describes a new form of sexuality, that of feminine sexuality. Here Lacan claims that the sliding of the subject among signification can stop with a form of an object that may be absent or present, the so-called small object a (*petit objet a*). This is connected with the maternal language and the lost phallus of the mother in contradistinction to the paternal language. Then he makes some formalizations upon signification by introducing the *raison* (reason) of the *master*, the *university*, the *analyst*, the *hysteric*, and the *capitalist*. He connects the use of that small object with the inclination or declination among the discourse, at last with his *Synthome*, or the synthe-

---

trace. This model emphasizes the plasticity of the human brain and thus the approach of the trace as not over-determined by its inscription, giving rise of a subject that acts in an autopoetic way by the creation of new traces from the inaugural traces. From a totally different perspective close to this kind of reconsolidation of memory, Derrida comments on Freud by saying Trace as memory is not a pure breaching that might be reappropriated at any time as simple presence; it is rather the ungraspable and invisible difference between breaches. We thus already know that psychic life is neither the transparency of meaning nor the opacity of force but the difference within the exertion of forces. As Nietzsche had already said that quantity becomes psyche and mneme through differences rather than through plenitudes will be continuously confirmed in the project itself, repetition adds no quantity of present force, no intensity; it reproduces the same impression – yet it has the power of breaching. "The memory of an experience (that is, its continuing operative power) depends on a factor which is called the magnitude of the impression and on the frequency with which the same impression is repeated" (Jacques Derrida, *Writing And Difference* (London: Routledge Classics, 1978), 201) Finally as to the phenomemenological approaches, the whole debate at least within this kind of perspective revolves around Merleau-Ponty and his considerations on the subject which always participates in the act of perceiving. The perceptual object is seen as a product of the encounter with the world. This led many scientists to experimentally explore brain function during the process of information assimilation and they found that the energy consumption of the brain is only 5% when perceiving and the other 95% is linked with the so-called "default mode of the brain", or the amount of the information that the retina can handle and therefore the brain ascribes a certain coherence among the information we perceive and so this coherence can be possibly linked with perceptual traces. In continuation, with phenomenology, there are the "bottom up" and "top down" theories. In the first, the trace is seen as an impression which remains in the mind; in the second, previously inscribed traces shape our perception. All these could be seen in comparison with the hallucinatory component of Freud, and the Lacanian "image" as a representation of a wishful activation.

sis of his circular particles of the *Boromenan Knot,* the *symbolic,* the *imaginary,* and the *real.*

It is known that Lacan interpreted Joyce; Derrida interpreted Antonin Artaud. What can we derive from those interpretations? We see first, for Lacan, the important issue of metrics in his analysis of the I-Schema and the canonical form of psychosis,[139] and for Derrida, the element of crudity or cruelty in the non-reducible Freudian psychodynamic of *Thanatos.*

And here we meet Donald Phillip Verene and his canons of speculative philosophy,[140] *Thanatos* as the Socratic. Those who, philosophizing rightly, are practicing to die (οι ορθώς φιλοσοφούντες αποθνήσκειν μελετώσι), either as the recollection of the Hegelian owl of Minerva and his theater, or as Vico's enlightenment of *sapienza* and *fantasia,* and finally his reading of James Joyce through Vico.[141] That part among signification is sublated to the whole process. That part is not something like a void; it is, rather, a self-relation or a self-reflection. It is not the part of the subject of not sensing, but works as the grounding of overcoming the double sense of in itself *(An sich).*

And this is our formalized (o)thereness, that "da" or "mitte", as the unifying part of the subject and the formalized Dehors. If we speculate on postmodern literature and, more specifically, on John Ashbery's "Self-Portrait in a Convex Mirror", it is because of the fact that American postmodern literature, starting from the haiku of Jack Kerouac, reflects the maxim of post-industrial America, and—more crucially—we have a return, a variable shift in form, the form of the writing subject. If for Harold Bloom the "Self-Portrait in a Convex Mirror" is T. S. Eliot's "The Waste Land", and John Ashbery a part of his Western canon, we can emphasize the fact of his strange Ashberian speculation. A probable

---

[139] Grigg Russell, *Lacan, Language, And Philosophy* (Albany, NY: State University of New York Press, 2008), 18-24: The discussion of Joyce some twenty years after the seminar on Schreber was not, as it happens, merely an occasion to explore further the issue of suppletion in relation to foreclosure. It resulted in nothing less than a reformulation of the way in which the differences between neurosis and psychosis should be approached and also contributed to an understanding of the difference between paranoia and schizophrenia ... The psychotic structure is then a transformation produced by the foreclosure of the Name-of-the-Father and the corresponding lack of phallic meaning of the neurotic structure. This thesis is apparent in the transformation of the R schema into the I schema.

[140] Donald Phillip Verene, *Speculative Philosophy* (Lanham, Maryland, Lexicom books, 2009), 1-11.

[141] Ibid., 93: The question Vico asks is how anything at all can be given for the mind. His view does not begin with something before the mind to know or to intend, but with how there is anything present for the mind and senses at all.

Levinasian non-univocity and non-reciprocity is given in a sublated way; the Other as well as death itself are the differential alters or mirror-reflections of the same poet, and therefore the writing subject.

In conclusion, the double reality of Gilles Deleuze and the real-semblance of Gungov, even more, give our final formalization. The Heideggerian possibility gives its place to actuality and the symbolic order of Lacan to the real-semblance. To return to medical philosophy, mirror neurons code the "why" of an action as reflecting the intentionality of the others; we meet the Heideggerian threefold of *existence(ze)*, *thrownness* and *fallenness*. If I am cheerful, the other possibly becomes cheerful; it is a matter of our mortal dwelling itself. And this very dwelling in our analysis is getting sublated. The cheerfulness is and was already "there". The activation of the "being cheerful" is an already existing actuality. But we do not presuppose a petit objet a or the cruelty of Derrida. It is me among the others, having a mutual understanding of everydayness and simultaneously co-transcending the maxim of an outer-extra signification: the formalizations of a Dehors.

Kant—and this could be a grounding against dogmatism—mainly bases his treatise upon pragmatism to certain founding principles that finally can be reduced to the reason (*Vernuft*), and freedom. This is the distinction upon the empirical and transcendental issues and the so-called *quaestio facti* and *quaestio iuris*. The general conception of justice may be "pure" and subjective but is always linked with its practical application to the various modes of experience. That is the main reason that Kant in his *Metaphysics of Ethics* clearly mentions that it cannot be founded upon anthropology, but it can be applied to it. Hegel taught us how we can overcome bad infinity, by his sublation (*Aufhebung*). But there is another more important feature that Hegel delivered to us: to think dialectically means to approach super-sensibility and, therefore, we can refer to the issue of an epistemological maxim and how it can be overcome.

Mainly with Heidegger and his Being as understanding and in our speculative phenomenological perception, we made all this circular route to "glare" this very fundamentality of poesies, the interiorizing and the eschatological exteriorizing, where the (o)therness of an exterior limit is "seen" as blockage or collapse of the eventual time of a horizon of dialectics (Ασυμβατότητα). The formalized (o)therness and the formalized Dehors as those modes of being as being, are partakers of that Dehors.

Chapter 4:
Objective and Subjective Medical Reasoning: An Overview

Introduction

We will start our chapter from a reverse side. We seek to explore and distinguish the various forms that philosophy of medicine follows so it meets the criteria of being a separate field. Beyond this, we investigate not the metaphysical, epistemological, or ethical presuppositions and foundations of the philosophy of medicine and how it interacts with them, but the basis of our analysis is that the philosophy of medicine, in order to define its subject matter and propose medical worldviews, creates for itself ways of cognition that demand the construction of terms, models, paradigms, and finally inquiries concerning its limits. The debate has arisen since the 70s, mainly in the US, but we will adopt Arthur Caplan's essay "Does the Philosophy of Medicine Exist?" (1992),as a starting point.[142] According to Caplan, there are three main lacks concerning the philosophy of medicine. First, to be a field it must be integrated into cognate areas of inquiry, to be a part of a discipline or set of disciplines. Second, there should be a canon in order to be a true field. Third, a discipline, if the philosophy of medicine is such, ought to create problems and puzzles which simultaneously define its theoretical and practical boundaries.[143] A primary response to Caplan is that the philosophy of medicine works upon the metaphysical and epistemological groundings of medical theory, experimentation, and practice. It contributes as a discipline to the general philosophy of science, providing conceptual frameworks and models of explanation, causation, and experimentation, as well as to bioethics, mainly on fundamental issues that arise in medical practice such as the concept of disease. Concerning its canon, there are plenty of academic journals devoted to the field and consequently proper academic literature that permits citations and references within the field and not through other fields. Finally, there are distinctive problems and questions that the philosophy of medicine pos-

---

[142] Claire Grignion and David Lefebre, *Medecins et philosophes une histoire* (Paris: CNRS editions, 2019), 10–14.
[143] A. L. Caplan, "Does the Philosophy of Medicine Exist?," *Theoretical Medicine*, no. 13 (1992): 67–77.

es, such as "What is the concept of disease", "What are the proper forms of medical reasoning and what are their limits?", "Is modern medicine a combination of evidence-based medicine and theoretical medicine?", and "Is medicine an art or strictly speaking a science?".[144]

4.1 From the Biomedical Model to a More Human-Based Approach, Towards a Paradigm Shift

Over the last years, there has been a great concern about the domination of the so-called biomedical model of medical practice that depends on biomedical sciences and their technologies, starting in the United States. The main critiques refer to the "disenchanted role of the physician"[145] or the "depersonalization and institutionalization of the healthcare system",[146] consequently affecting the quality of care and broadening the debate over the approach of medical practice and the doctor-patient relationship. The counterargument to the biomedical approach is that it does not account much for the particularity of the patient (treating *a patient* or *this patient*), especially on the level of experiencing his condition, for example the sentiments of pain, suffering, anxiety, etc., and how they affect the progression of his problem and the healing process. Furthermore, there are external factors affecting the patient, e.g., social, cultural, etc., and internal such as the brute facts and moral and aesthetic information of the patient on the process of reasoning and in the doctor-patient relationship, a theory developed by Eric Cassell.[147] In this respect, two separate models of medical reasoning were established: the biomedical or objective, and the humanistic or subjective models. These models differ as to their metaphysical and epistemological foundations. Through these preliminary considerations, it is shown how a concern, based on real and adequately justified problems, leads to a general rethinking of the models of reasoning in medicine and the creation of new worldviews or paradigms.

---

[144] For a more detailed list of problems and questions that philosophy of medicine poses see: David Låg Tomasi, *Medical Philosophy A Philosophical Analysis Of Patient Self-Perception In Diagnostics And Therapy* (Stuttgart: Ibidem Press, 2016), 3.

[145] F. J. Ingelfinger, "Medicine: meritorious or meretricious," *Science, no.* 200 (1978): 942–946.

[146] S. M. Glick, "Humanistic medicine in a modern age," *New England Journal of Medicine, no.* 304 (1981): 1036–1038.

[147] Cf. Eric Cassell, *The Nature Of Suffering And The Goals Of Medicine* (New York: Oxford University Press, 1991).

Thomas Kuhn, in his book *The Structure of Scientific Revolutions* (1962), follows the general aspects of non-linearity in history. Scientific progress is not a progressive accumulation of facts and data, but rather is paradigm-driven. The aim of the book is to present a different concept of science than is often presented with the processing of historical data. Historians should have two main tasks. First, they explain by whom and when a scientific fact, law, or theory was invented or discovered. Second, they have to explain the congeries of error and superstition that did not allow modern science to proceed. Scientific development is done by posing crucial questions about phenomena. Observation and experience then restrict the range of the admissible scientific belief. The transition points in science with special characteristics are mentioned in the book as scientific revolutions. Each of them produced a subsequent shift in the problems available for scientific scrutiny and transformed the world within which scientific work is done.

How does a single paradigm work? It works through an esoteric, built-in mechanism that ensures the relaxation of the restrictions that bound research whenever the paradigm from which they are derived ceases to function effectively. There are three foci for factual scientific investigation: first, the class of facts the paradigm uses to reveal the nature of things, second, the usual class of factual determination diverges from those facts which are without much intrinsic interest and can be directly correlated with predictions from the paradigm theory, and finally, experimentation.

Normal science research can be characterized as puzzle-solving. Puzzles are a special category of problems that can serve to test ingenuity or skills. Usually, the problems that are undertaken are based on paradigms; the others may be rejected as metaphysical. There is always some kind of motivation among scientists to solve a problem that has not been solved so well. There are many rules in the normal scientific tradition that provide a great deal of information about commitments that scientists derive from their paradigms. For instance, the scientist must be concerned to understand the world and to extend the precision and scope with which it has been ordered.

4.2 Different Worldviews/Paradigms and Different Foundations

According to Diederik Aerts et al. in their *World Views From Fragmentation to Integration* (2007), the first of seven basic elements of a worldview is the reply to the questions "What is the nature of our world?" and "How is it structured and how does it function?".[148] Of course, they speak about the metaphysical positions that are necessary for the foundation of a certain worldview. The biomedical model holds in its core the position of mechanistic monism. There are different kinds of monism, like priority monism, which targets concrete objects and counts basic tokens, connected with the doctrine of the whole as prior to its parts. There is also existence monism, which targets concrete objects and counts by tokens, and which is the analysis of a doctrine of existence of exactly one object token. They all share the assumption of oneness of an existence of one ultimate substance that constitutes the word. Monism is distinguished from dualism, which speaks about two ultimate substances (usually in the philosophy of medicine we refer to the revolution of Cartesian dualism that separates the mind as non-physical thinking substance—*res cogitans*—and the body as substance extended in space—*res extensa*), and pluralism, which refers to three or more substances. Finally, nihilism posits that all values are baseless and nothing can be known or communicated.

The ultimate substance for the biomedical model is matter. This conception is connected with physicalism or materialism, but the second is an older manifestation. The term mechanical or mechanistic is related to the position that the patient is a collection of parts; each part has its appropriate functions. The oneness of the patient is the result of the combination of these parts, like a machine.[149]

The metaphysical presupposition, which is strongly associated with physicalism of the biomedical model, is reductionism. Reductionism may be theoretical, and it involves the reduction of terms of different theories to one. Secondly, as ontological, it investigates the ordering of phenomena and claims that the higher order is determined by a lower order. And finally, as methodological, which is close to ontological, it speaks for a

---

[148]   Aerts, Diederik et al. 2007. *World Views from Fragmentation to Integration*. Ebook. Clément Vidal and AlexanderRiegler.https://www.researchgate.net/publiccation/244529051_Worldviews_From_Fragmentation_to_Integration.

[149]   James Marcum, *Humanizing Modern Medicine an Introductory Philosophy of Medicine* (Springer, 2008), 19.

complex or higher-order structure which is constituted by more simple or lower-order structures; e.g., the intermediate metabolic pathways are conceived of in terms of their separate molecular components.[150]

As regards the representatives of the humanistic or humane model in medicine we have two large categories concerning the recognition and appreciation of the biomedical model. The large majority recognizes the valuable technical advantages of the biomedical model that contributed to medical theory and practice. There is also a minority that completely rejects it. One basic counterargument is that since mechanistic monism presupposes one ultimate substance—i.e., matter—on that basis it equates the mind with the brain. This equation also involves patient psychology and social factors as separate and non-reducible in diagnosis, treatment, and recovery. Humanistic models like the biopsychosocial model proposed by Engel, or the model of narrative reasoning, emphasize the role that experience of an illness plays in the prognosis and therapeutic process.

The humanistic model is based on dualism or holism as its metaphysical grounding. This dualism is not only the Cartesian interactionism of mind/body as *res-cogitans/res-extensa*, but a more extended view of it, which, as briefly mentioned above, accounts for the patient's environmental, social, and cultural context. As a consequence, the humanistic model seeks to explore the interaction of the patient with themselves, their family, society, and healthcare practitioners.[151]

On a practical level, the patient is not approached solely as a diseased body which a reductionist approach would treat, but as a person, as a particularity with a certain subjective experience of his illness, with relevant existential or religious concerns, etc. At last, we have a variable shift in the doctor-patient relationship. It is no more the impersonal and strictly scientific relationship, based on interpretation of objective clinical or statistical data and implementation of protocols of diagnosis, treatment, and prognosis, but rather a relationship based on interpersonal active communication, which moves to the sphere of the patient's subjective experience and concerns. "The physician can understand the patient's illness which is an essential part of the humanistic approach to illness".[152]

---

[150]   Ibid., 26.
[151]   Ibid., 20.
[152]   I. Switankowsky, "Dualism and its importance for medicine," *Theoretical Medicine,* no. 21 (2001), 567–580.

The metaphysical presupposition of the humanistic model is emergentism. Emergentism comes from the Latin verb *emergo*, which means to appear, to escape, to rise up.[153] As a term in philosophy, it comes from J. S. Mill in his *System of Logic* (1875). According to Mill, most of the effects and laws in nature follow the principle "composition of causes". In some cases, this principle is not valid. For example, in the chemical equation $H^{2+}O^2 = H^2O$, the product cannot be seen as a simple sum of the reactants. The component substances that react are "mere physical agents".[154] Mill calls the laws fulfilling such instances "heteropathic" laws.[155] Later on, Mill's student and follower G. H. Lewes will call the "composition of causes" "resultants" and the "heteropathic events" "emergents". [156]

Emergentism also arose in the debate of the late 19th and early 20th century among reductive mechanists—who speak about ordering (e.g., higher-order phenomena that recomposed of lower-order phenomena)— and the "component theory" of the vitalists. The debate was about how the properties of a complex structure or system are composed of the properties of its parts. C. D. Broad, in his *Mind and Its Place in Nature* (1925), tries to give an alternative reply. In distinction with the oneness of the reductionism that conceives of the world as homogenous, Broad states that reality is structured in formations of a different order. The different order presupposes a different organizational complexity; the units that compose each order are found in lower orders. This process obeys different kinds of laws: trans-ordinal laws that connect properties of adjacent orders and intra-ordinal laws that hold between properties within the same order. These laws are irreducible to each other and thus are fundamental emergent laws, or can be taken as metaphysical brute facts.[157]

Two main aspects of emergentism are *determinism* and *unpredictability*. Following Achim Stephan, the first is connected with synchronic emergentism, which means that the properties and behavior of a system are nomologically dependent on its microstructure. An alteration of a

153 "Latin Definition for Emergo" Ladict, last modified January 29, 2020, http://latin-dicti onary.net/definition/19005/emergo-emergere-emersi-emersus
154 John Stuart Mill, System of Logic Ratiocinative and Inductive. Collected Works, Volumes 7 and 8 (Toronto: University of Toronto Press, 1996), 371.
155 Ibid., 374.
156 Brian P. McLaughlin, *The Rise and Fall of British Emergentism* (Beckermann, A., Flohr, H., & Kim, J, 1992), 65.
157 C. D. Broad, *The Mind and its Place in Nature* (London: Kegan Paul, Trench, Trubner & Co., 1925), 23, 77–78.

system cannot be accomplished without an alteration to its microstructure, something that nowadays is called *supervenience*. *Unpredictability* is in relation to *diachronic* emergentism. This theory proposes that under the same initial conditions the same events will happen and the same structures will emerge.[158]

4.3 Objectivity Versus Subjectivity

Following the general division between the two main models of medical reasoning, we now refer in detail to their epistemological assumptions. Biomedical practitioners subscribe to an objective way of thinking. Objectivity means that knowledge is valid in every context, social, cultural, etc., and does not take into account one's particular values. Our emotions and intuitions can distort our objective view of the world. The final target of objective thinking in medicine is to assure a patient's safety by eliminating mistakes in medical cognition or, broadly, to best obtain and substantiate knowledge. Humanistic or humane practitioners follow a subjective way of reasoning. Intuitions, values, and virtues are important for the knower—e.g., the patient's narrative of the illness, or the subjective meaning of a practitioner in his/her healing role.[159]

Objectivity and subjectivity in medicine do not refer solely to the groundings of the two models above. They are also crucial for the understanding of medicine as art or as science and if it is based on a value-free or value-laden relationship. According to T. V. Cunningham,

> When understood in terms of objectivity and subjectivity, the debate over whether medicine is a science comes down to whether medicine is "purely objective" and aims at the accumulation of objective knowledge, or whether it includes an inherently "subjective" component. This "subjective" component has been rendered in terms of personal values in the debate over the scientificity of medicine. In this way, we see the interplay between the value-free/value-laden distinction and the distinction between objectivity and subjectivity, in that medicine is an art if it aims at understanding patients' subjective knowledge of illness in terms that are patently laden with the patient's values. Likewise, medicine is understood as a science in

---

[158] A. Stephan, "Varieties of emergentism," *Evolutions and Cognition*, no. 5 (1999): 49–59.
[159] James Marcum, *Humanizing Modern Medicine An Introductory Philosophy Of Medicine* (Springer, 2008), 97.

as much as it aims to understand patients' diseases in objective terms, meaning those that are disconnected from the values of particular patients and clinicians.[160]

There are two main basic theories of objectivity, rationalism and empiricism. Rationalists argue that our analytic or a priori knowledge is produced through our innate mind's action and cannot be directly experienced. Knowledge that comes from our senses can be corrupted or deceiving. There are three fundamental claims of rationalism. The first is *the intuition/deduction thesis* which deals with our beliefs and propositions in particular subject areas. The second is the *innate knowledge thesis*: we have knowledge of some truths in a subject area as an intrinsic characteristic of our rational nature. The last is the *innate concept thesis*: we employ concepts in particular subject areas as an intrinsic characteristic of our rational nature. Empiricism focuses upon *a posteriori* or synthetic knowledge and poses that knowledge is obtained only through sense experience. The *empiricist thesis* is: We have no source of knowledge, or we do not employ any concepts in particular subject areas other than our sense experience.[161]

4.4 Objective Thinking Based on Statistics

The two main statistical methods used in objective medical reasoning are Bayesian statistics and frequentist statistics. The probability distributions that Bayesian statistics construct are for unknown quantities of interest based on the given data. Their main thesis is that unknown quantities, such as population means and proportions, obey probability distributions. The probability distribution for a population proportion reflects knowledge of belief which is prior to us, before we add the knowledge which comes from our data. In Bayesian analysis, researchers estimate a prior distribution for the event of interest in order to run the analysis of a data set. This prior distribution may be based on a variety of external evidence that includes controlled and uncontrolled studies, case reports, and expert opinions. A pivotal difficulty is how to decide on the prior distribution. This is likely to have an effect on the conclusions of the study, yet it may be a subjective synthesis of the available information,

---

[160]   Cf. Thomas V. Cunningham, "Objectivity, Scientificity, And The Dualist Epistemology Of Medicine," in *Classification, Disease and Evidence, History, 1 Philosophy And Theory Of The Life Sciences*. (Dordrecht: Springer Science+Business Media, 2001).

[161]   Markie, Peter, "Rationalism vs. Empiricism," *The Stanford Encyclopedia of Philosophy* (Fall 2017 Edition), Edward N. Zalta (ed.), URL=<https://plato.stanford.edu/archives/fall2017/entries/rationalism-empiricism/>.

so the same data analyzed by different investigators could lead to different conclusions. Another difficulty is that Bayesian methods may lead to intractable computational problems.[162] There are also benefits from Bayesian statistics, on a practical level. According to Lewis and Wear, since they have decreased the error rate in comparison with the frequentist method, it is possible that a clinical trial in progress can be terminated earlier; therefore, fewer patients will be exposed to ineffective or harmful therapy. Finally, with Bayesian statistics we can determine the possibility of a particular event—e.g., the efficacy of a drug.

Frequentist methods regard the population value as a fixed, unvarying (but unknown) quantity, without a probability distribution. Frequentists then calculate confidence intervals for this quantity, or significance tests of hypotheses concerning it. This is very different from the Bayesian view of probability—being a degree of belief or knowledge about the unknown. Thus, this permits us to have knowledge of a future event by the combination of past data.[163]

Frequentist statistics first form a null hypothesis. For example, between two groups of treatment—A and B—there will not be significant statistical difference. Together with the null hypothesis, an alternative hypothesis is formed, which claims that there will be a difference. Therefore, if our calculations lead us to reject the null hypothesis, the treatment used in group B will be more efficient than group A. There are at least two problems with Frequentist statistics in medical practice. First, we do not have direct proof that the alternative hypothesis is true. According to Lewis and Wears, "there may be many alternative hypotheses different from the original one that might have been accepted based on this evidence had they been proposed." Second, frequentist statistics usually deal with populations and not individual patients. Thus, for example, we cannot have the probability of *this* patient dying tonight; we can only have access to data such as what percentage of patients with similar statistical data will die tonight.[164]

[162] Bland J. Martin, Douglas G. Altman "Bayesians and frequentists," *BMJ* (1998): 317–1151.
[163] Perkins, Jan and Wang, Daniel "A Comparison of Bayesian and Frequentist Statistics as Applied in a Simple Repeated Measures Example," *Journal of Modern Applied Statistical Methods*, no. 3 (2004).
[164] R. J. Lewis, R. L. Wears, "An introduction to the Bayesian analysis of clinical trials," *Annals of Emergency Medicine*, no. 22 (1999): 1328–1336.

4.5 Objective Thinking as Evidence-Based Medicine

Evidence-based medicine as a method or reasoning took its name from a movement (with that name) that was started in the early 1990s by a group of epidemiologists at McMaster University in Hamilton, Ontario. The main doctrine of the group was that medical practitioners should attain greater reliance on the current form of published research, with emphasis on clinical trials. The value and reliability of evidence should be considered in a form of hierarchy, with trial data taking the first or higher and authoritative position, and clinical judgment and mechanical reasoning, secondary or lower, due to the latter's unreliability.[165] The notion of a hierarchy of evidence was later dismissed by some members of the movement, and they proposed an alternative definition: "Evidence based medicine is the conscientious, explicit, and judicious use of current best evidence in making decisions about the care of individual patients."[166] The terms "judicious" and "best evidence" seem to generalize and float and these presuppositions could fit in every clinical context, even before the hierarchy of the evidence-based movement or even before the method of clinical trials.

Evidence-based medicine has a considerable limitation that concerns both the method of clinical trials, as well as the same medical practice. As to the clinical trials, an important issue is that of the *unrepresentativeness of trial subjects*. Well-structured clinical trials, in most cases, define their preconditions of participation. Usually there is the limitation of age (exact range), the presence of another disease is also accounted for, and a certain range of clinical or biochemical criteria is implemented. Consequently, only a minority of those with the condition are recruited.[167] Secondly, *long-term therapy* can also affect the reliability of a trial. There are several cases of patients receiving long-term therapy, and even lifetime therapy or combinations of therapies, that in the progress of science may have changed, and the data available from clini-

---

[165]   Evidence-Based Medicine Working Group, "Evidence-based medicine: a new approach to teaching the practice of medicine," *JAMA*, no. 17 (1992): 2420–25.

[166]   D. L. Sackett, W. M. Rosenberg, J. A. Gray, R. B. Haynes, and W. S. Richardson, "Evidence-Based Medicine: What it Is and What it Isn't," *British Medical Journal*, no. 312 (1996): 71–72.

[167]   P. Y. Lee, K. P. Alexander, B. G. Hammill, et al., "Representation of elderly persons and women in published randomized trials of acute coronary syndromes," *JAMA*, no. 286 (2001): 708–13.

cal trial evidence may be limited to a period of 5-10 years.[168] *Comorbidity* also plays an important role. Comorbid patients are usually excluded from the clinical trials; their condition in most cases can seriously affect the results of a trial due to the fact that one condition may overlap with the results of another or demand a combination of pharmaceutical treatments.[169] There are cases in which physicians try to balance between *statistical* and *clinical* significance. The priority of the p-value of 0.05% as statistically significant in most trials may create a buffer zone between those who, according to the trial, will have a beneficial or harmful therapeutic effect. In clinical practice, the particularity of the patient or of a group of patients determines whether to proceed with a given action, so we can speak for an opposition of the two methods of significance.[170] Finally, there is the issue of misleading results in clinical trials. Bias can occur from improper statistical analysis concerning the methods used for the trial and non-publication of important statistical results, mainly those referring to negative effects of a protocol or drug. More importantly, trials funded by pharmaceutical companies should be regarded with suspicion due to possible conflicts of interest.

In medical practice, there are two main biases on the role of clinical trials; the first is the bias of *the easily measurable*. While outcome measures such as mortality, morbidity, and cost effectiveness are easily accessed and measurable, other equally important factors are excluded and not easily quantified, such as the quality of the care, a patient's experience, the respect of human dignity, and the contributions to the knowledge base. The second is the bias in *commissioned research*. The issue concerns the directions of medical research in general, and what its motor is. Is it scientists who are engaged in cutting-edge research or the sponsors and companies that regulate funding according to what they deem a priority?[171]

[168] X. Rossello, S. J. Pocock, D. G. Julian. "Long-term use of cardiovascular drugs: challenges for research and for patient care," *Journal of the American College of Cardiology* no. 66 (2015): 1273–85.
[169] H. G. Van Spall, A. Toren, A. Kiss, et al., "Eligibility criteria of randomized controlled trials published in high-impact general medical journals: a systematic sampling review," *JAMA*, no. 297 (2007): 1233–40.
[170] MIAMI Trial Research Group, "Long-term prognosis after early intervention with metoprolol in suspected acute myocardial infarction: experiences from the MIAMI Trial," *J Intern Med*, no. 230 (2001): 233–37.
[171] Sheridan, Desmond J., and Desmond G. Desmond G, "Achievements and Limitations of Evidence-Based Medicine," *Journal of the American College of Cardiology*, no. 2 (2001).

4.6 Subjective Thinking

Generally humanistic or humane practitioners recognize that laboratory data and clinical observations are important or even necessary in practice, although they are not sufficient. According to them, treatment demands a subjective personalized knowledge which is critical for treating *this* patient instead of *a* patient described in clinical statistical data or trials.

Eric Cassell argues that in medical practice, physicians get a narrow understanding of objectivity while subjectivity prevails. Imagine you feel feverish, he says. You are achy and have cold sweats. You feel ill. If you go to a physician and he takes your temperature, then "the reading on the clinical thermometer is an objective measurement of an elevation of body temperature. The feeling of feverishness is subjective because a feeling can only be experienced by the subject." This is one sense of what it means to be subjective; it is to feel a certain way, which can only be felt by you, the subject. There are also three senses, associated with subjectivity. The first concerns the *ideas* about the *way you feel*. The second refers to the subjective way that we resonate about our state of affairs—i.e., subjective feeling. The last is connected with the statement and its meaning. "Your *statement* that you feel feverish is also considered subjective. What the words *mean* is not something outside observers can hold in common". Hence, they are subjective too.[172]

Cassell holds a belief of value-laden medicine. For him there are three kinds of information about sick persons: brute facts, moral, and aesthetic. All three are necessary for the work of the clinician. Brute facts can be seen as an objective form of information needed to evaluate the patient's physical condition, the degree of the problem's progression, etc., although it is not sufficient. The patient's moral and aesthetic sensibilities are those which build a better understanding of the patient, and thus help to reveal the subjective feeling of suffering. Only when the physician is aware of this information can he originally care for and assist the patient in the healing process.[173]

On the basis of personal knowledge, Cassell proceeds to emphasize the importance of values in medical knowledge. Applying medical science to particular patients mandates thinking in terms of values as much

---

[172]   Eric Cassell, *The Nature of Suffering and The Goals of Medicine* (New York: Oxford University Press), 171.
[173]   Ibid., 226.

as in terms of objective facts about the body, Cassell asserts.[174] There are at least five sources of values needed for substantiating medical knowledge: the values society places on health and illness, the goals of medical care in general, physicians' personal and professional values, people's individual values, and the values that undergird the operations of a system as a complex unity or whole.[175]

Psychiatrist George L. Engel proposed the biopsychosocial model of thinking. In his article "The need for a new medical model: A challenge for biomedicine" (1977), he criticized the dominant model of disease, the so-called biomedical model. This model, having molecular biology as its basic scientific discipline, conceives of disease as deviating from the norm of measurable somatic variables. The social, psychological, and behavioral dimensions of illness are not part of its subject matter. As for the behavioral aberrations, the biomedical model seeks to explain them on the basis of disordered somatic (biochemical or neurophysiological) processes. Concerning the above, the biomedical model has a reductionist foundation which views complex phenomena as derived from a single primary principle and a mind-body dualism that separates the mental from the somatic. Thinking about mental disease, Engel states that the biomedical dogma permits only two alternatives: the *reductionist*, which says that all behavioral phenomena must be regarded in terms of physico-chemical principles, and the *exclusionist*, which mentions the possibility of something that cannot be explained to be excluded from the category of disease.[176]

Engel proposes three main topics that the biopsychosocial model should focus on and correct in regard to the biomedical model: first, the *recognition of complex causation*: "The biomedical defect constitutes but one factor among many, the complex interaction of which ultimately may culminate in active disease or manifest illness"[177]; second, the *recognition of various levels of activity*: "how [a disease such as diabetes with attendant polyuria, polydipsia, polyphagia, and weight loss, confirmed by laboratory documentation of relative insulin deficiency, is experienced, reported by, and affects any one individual requires] consideration of psychological, social and cultural factors, not to mention other concur-

---

[174]   Ibid., 178.
[175]   Ibid., 184.
[176]   George L. Engel, "The Need for a New Medical Model: A Challenge for Biomedicine," *Science*, no. 4286, (1971): 129–36.
[177]   Ibid.

rent or complicating biological factors"[178]; and last, *recognition of the individual variability of a disease,* which "reflects as much, psychological, social, and cultural factors as it does quantitative variations in the specific biochemical defect".[179]

Laurence Foss, in his book *The End of Modern Medicine: Biomedical Science Under a Microscope* (2002), calls for an alternative model of medical thinking in which information can be incorporated in medical practice. This model is called "infomedical". Foss explores the consequences of the conjunction of the body, mind, and information. For Foss there are special carriers of our sociocultural inheritance called "memes". Memes are self-replicating psychological information units.[180] Foss investigates the case of anorexia nervosa. Anorexia nervosa is generally linked with the social norms reproduced by the mass media concerning the ideal body shape. In a way, those who suffer from this disease always have the self-image of someone who is never "that thin". A valuable remark is that anorexics can lose weight beyond the minimum required to sustain basal metabolism. Foss says about this:

> And the conjectured reason is that the mind-brain, through the messages it sends (transduced via messenger molecules), can actually alter the metabolism in such a way that the calories are burned up as fuel instead of stored as fat. An image or belief, a "memetic" vector, interacts with metabolism, the offspring of genetic instructions. ... The infomedical conclusion is clear. The anorexic can make herself ill or well depending not solely on what she does or doesn't eat but also on the signals she sends to herself (and those she processes from her culture). In other words, depending on how she (and her culture) programs herself. Her behavior is the synergistic commingling of her memetic *and* genetic programming. [181]

There is a mechanism for Foss that transfers information among parts of the organism and between the organism and its environment. He reformulates the second law of thermodynamics as the second law of psychothermodynamics in which the universal dynamic is vitalistic and autopoietic.[182] Finally, he speaks about a subjectified objectivity; for him, "the object is subject, the patient is an agent, each possessing some limited degree of autonomy".[183]

---

[178]   Ibid.
[179]   Ibid.
[180] . Laurence Foss, *The End of Modern Medicine Biomedical Science Under a Microscope* (New York: State University of New York Press, Albany, 2002), 142.
[181]   Ibid., 144.
[182]   Ibid., 233.
[183]   Ibid., 242.

The final form of subjective medical reasoning that we will discuss is *narrative reasoning*. This type aims to access personal information on the level of disruption of a patient's life by an illness. It is concerned with the meaning and significance of the patient's illness story, in distinction to the biomedical model that focuses on objective clinical data that define the nature of the disease itself. The narrative reasoning investigates the process of getting ill, getting better, and coping with illness within the wider narratives of people's lives. It is a holistic approach to illness and may uncover alternative or new diagnostic and therapeutic options. Narratives are methods that address existential qualities, such as inner hurt, despair, hope, grief, and moral pain which frequently accompany, or even define, people's illnesses.[184]

Cheryl Mattingly identifies three features of narrative reasoning in medicine. The first concerns the motives that trigger a patient's story in terms of actions and their consequences. The next step is the construction of a patient's social world. The practitioner can now understand the effects of the illness on the social level, how it affects the patient's everydayness and sociality—e.g., the relation with his/her relatives and his/her social environment—as well as the patient's existential or even transcendent concerns, if we refer to the realms beyond our world and situations of near-death experience, etc. The final feature involves the probable and possible, rather than the determinant and necessary, as in logical biomedical reasoning: "Narrative is needed to contemplate the world and its complexities and to decipher how one should navigate one's way in it, for narrative is built on surprise, chance, contingency and the anomalous event".[185]

Gadamer, in his *Enigma of Health*[186], states that illnesses could be seen as a "revolt", when something does not work properly. The nature of health is to sustain its own proper balance and proportion. He uses the term *Gegenstand* (object) which resists (*Widerstand*). Contrary to illness, health is not revealed through investigation but rather is something that always escapes our attention. We are not constantly vigilant about health as we are about illness. Gadamer claims that beyond the bodily problem in which the illness is manifested, there is always a problem of the soul. In a manner, the body is linked with life, and the soul is what animates.

[184]   Trisha Greenhalgh, Brian Hurwitz. "Why study narrative?" *BMJ*, no. 318 (1999): 48.
[185]   Cheryl Mattingly, "In search of the good: narrative reasoning in clinical practice," *MedicaAnthropology*, (1999): 273–97.
[186]   Hans-Georg Gadamer, *The Enigma of health the Art of Healing in a Scientific Age*, trans. Jason Gaiger and Nicolas Walker. (Cambridge: Polity Press, 1996), 93–114.

Gadamer, in a reference to Hegel, concludes that spirit is both the body and that which animates it.

For modern science, to objectify means to measure the natural phenomena connected with health and illness, and, in our time, this measurement does not take place in the eyes of the patient but through specialized medical instruments. Gadamer makes a passage through Platonic philosophy and the two kinds of measure, *metron* and *metrion*, in order to speak for the inner measure which is proper to a self-sustaining living whole. Health is thus a condition of harmony, of an appropriate state of internal measure. Illness, on the other hand, is seen as a disturbance of the harmony of the balanced sentiments of feeling well and our active way of interacting with the world. So, there are two different forms of measure: one of science and the other of the totality of our being-in-the-world. Here appears the distinction between treatment (*Behandlung*), which is equal to handling people with the care of the hand that feels and touches, and the objective state of specialized medical measurements by instruments. Gadamer uses the term "inappropriate" (*ungemäß*) for the application of rules on the basis of prior measurements that we naturally do. He continues with a second distinction between two forms of measure: the first, a natural form of measure in which the things bear in themselves, and a second, which describes how the patient feels ill. Furthermore, when we speak about *Behandlen*, or *palapare* (palpus), the good doctor should carefully and responsively feel the patient's body to detect the signs which can confirm or reject the subjective location which is the patient's subjective feeling of pain which in a way resists and establishes a disruption of the harmony which accompanies health. This form of palliative care also means not to impose any authority or force on the patient so as to make him/her accept something against his/her will. It is rather to recognize the other in its otherness, and the meaning of the dialogue is to humanize the fundamentally unequal doctor-patient relation. Treatment, or *therapeia,* in Greek, has the meaning of service, and this service should be not only effective against illness, but also accepted by the patient. Health and recovery are not a condition that one feels oneself; they are a condition of being-in-the-world, of being together with one's fellow human beings. We are partners, part (and here Gadamer recalls Husserl) of a life world which supports us all.

4.7 Doctor-Patient Relationship in the Information Age

There are various conceptualizations of the basic models of the doctor-patient relationship; we will only refer to two of them which remain quite popular. The first is proposed by Thomas Szasz and Marc Hollender and the second by Ezekiel and Linda Emanuel. We will proceed from the general aspects of the characteristics and the interaction that may shape this kind of relationship, to then analyze how this relationship is affected in the information age.

Szasz and Hollender propose a three-part scheme.[187] The first conceptualization is the model of activity-passivity. This is the oldest proposed model. Today it is mainly linked with medical interventions like anesthesia, acute trauma, coma, and delirium, cases in which the patient is not in a position to interact with the doctor and demand medical management. The prototype of this model is the parent-infant relationship. As the parent aims for the protection and proper growth of the infant, the doctor aims for the rehabilitation of the health and well-being of the patient unable to interact. The second model is that of clinical guidance. This model is based on the cooperation of the doctor and the patient. The patient is not in such a desperate condition as those listed above; it may be an acute inflammation, which is the most common in medical practice. The patient feels anxiety, pain, and distress from his condition, and on the other hand he is conscious and has feelings and aspirations of his own, so he is willing to cooperate. This model has as a prototype in the parent-adolescent relationship. In this case the two participants are both active and contribute to the relationship. But as the parent "holds power", in the same way the doctor will offer guidance and leadership and expect cooperation from the other participants. Thus, the patient is expected to "look up to" and obey his doctor; furthermore, there is no place for questioning or disagreement with the order he receives. The third model is that of mutual participation; this model conceives of the two participants as equal. It is based on at least three presuppositions: first, that the participants have approximately equal power; second, that they are mutually interdependent; and third, that they engage in activity that will be satisfying to both. This model is more appropriate for patients who can take care of themselves (at least to a certain extent) and can be compatible, for example, with the management of chronic health diseases like diabetes

---

[187]   T. S Szasz and M. H. Hollender, "The Basic Models of the Doctor-Patient Relationship," *Archives of Internal Medicine* 97, (1956): 585–92.

and chronic heart disease. It demands more complex psychological and social organization, so it should not be utilized with children or the mentally deficient.

Emanuel and Emanuel outline four models of the doctor-patient interaction.[188] The first model is the paternalistic model. This model, often called the parental or priestly model, favors the role of the doctor. The doctors use their skills to define the patient's conditions, and—with the belief that there are some shared objective criteria determining what is best— proceeds to tests and treatments that will restore the patient's health or mitigate pain. Or, to put it differently, the doctor collects all the information needed and presents it to the patient, encouraging him to consent to an intervention. This model seemingly does not much account for the patient's autonomy.

The second model is the informative model, sometimes called the consumer model. In this case the doctor provides the patient with all the relevant information and the patient selects the intervention. The information provided by the doctor has the form of facts, so it may be the state of disease, the form of diagnostic and therapeutic interventions, the possible lack of knowledge, and the risks and benefits. The patient decides according to his values; the values of the doctor do not play any role and he is seen more as a specialized technician who will clarify the facts. In this model the conception of patient autonomy is patient control over medical decision-making.

The third model is the interpretive model; this model's goal is a doctor-patient interaction that elucidates the patient's values and goals. As in the informative model, the doctor provides the patient with the appropriate information, but here also helps the patient clarify his values to determine what kind of medical interventions best realize those values. According to this model the patient has no fixed value, so the doctors should reconstruct the patient's aspirations as they together find the best solution. The conception of the patient's autonomy in this model is equal to the patient's self-understanding.

The fourth is the deliberative model. In this model the doctors aim to suggest why certain health-related values are more worthy than others. In this way, the doctor recognizes that some elements of morality are not related to the patient's disease and the scope of their relationship. It is a form of moral deliberation in which doctor and patient judge the worthi-

---

[188]   Ezekiel J. Emanuel and Linda L. Emanuel, "The Physician-Patient Relationship," JAMA 267, no. 16 (1992): 2221–26.

ness and importance of the health-related issues. The patient's autonomy here is equal to moral self-development.

Deborah Lupton investigates the new status of patients and care-givers interacting on digital platforms by sharing their personal narratives or experience of illness, and also seeking health-related information or providing advice and promoting their services.[189] The general concept of these platforms is for patients to promote their own health by accessing relevant information and monitoring their health from electronic health records and from wearable devices that register vital parameters for their condition. In this way they can take responsibility for self-management and possibly lessen the burden on the health care system. The other, also important, issue is that these platforms aim to promote the image of the digitally engaged patient who becomes more knowledgeable about his health and illness and provides information to other patients and health care practitioners.

Lupton argues that, beyond the general benefits, the patients be-come part of a "digital patient experience economy". This is related to the extreme commoditization of the patient's experience. Lupton also speaks for an economy of prosumption (the combination of content consumption and production in web 2.0). Patients do not offer or receive financial compensation. The value of prosumers is non-commercial; the exchange value of their data is directed to non-profit organizations and at last possibly to commercial entities that can benefit from their use. This can be seen from the fact that over the last years there was an increase in the publication of mass-market journals devoted to health which gradual-ly led today to all these digital platforms. Concerning the digital plat-forms, there are strong ethical implications, since the patients may in most cases give a form of consent when they upload information, but they do not have any access to the information management. The infor-mation is intellectual property of the website owner and can be used and sold to insurance companies, pharmaceutical companies, and various stakeholders and policy-makers.

Marion Ball and Jennifer Lillis describe at least three characteris-tics of modern e-health consumers.[190] First, they seek convenience; many of them are well-educated and avoid wasting time in long queues for

---

[189]   Deborah Lupton, "The commodification of patient opinion: the digital patient experi-ence economy in the age of big data," *Sociology of Health and Ilness* 36, no. 5 (2014): 856–69.

[190]   Marion J. Ball and Jennifer Lillis, "E-Health: transforming the physician/patient relationship, " *International Journal of Medical Informatics* 61, (2001):1–10.

appointments. Second, they wish to have control of their own health or at least play a significant role in it, so they seek internet resources to supplement the information they receive from their physicians. Third, they demand a wide variety of choices for every service and product they require; this is reinforced by the fact that more and more people are willing to use alternative therapies, such as acupuncture or nutritional supplements. Ball also refers to the administrative efficiency that computerization in health care delivered, like the reduction of waste of time and paper, since all the necessary documents are shared directly in a digital form, the improvement of outcomes through online prescription systems, and cost reduction by the use of simple automatic processes. She also makes some propositions for the doctor-patient relationship in the information age to follow a better path. Ball suggests that physicians recommend appropriate websites to their patients to prevent them from relying on faulty medical information; for example, in the US, reputable medical websites display the HONcode logo. Doctors' recommendations are seen as the most important factor in building consumer trust in online information. Furthermore, they can create a website (or a social media page) to provide information, schedule appointments online, create bulletin boards, and provide explanations of their services. Ball insists that doctors should exchange emails with their patients; since as a form of written communication they last and can be read at any time. This method of communication can reduce frustration and save time.

Miriam McMullan proposes three scenarios concerning the doctor-patient relation in the information age.[191] The first scenario is health professional-centered. The doctor may feel that his knowledge and authority are threatened; thus, he responds defensively and asserts his expert opinion; he can have a short consultation and authoritatively direct the patient towards his choice of action. The second scenario is more patient-centered; in this scenario, the doctor and patient collaborate. Patients may not have time to search for information regarding their health problems; on the other hand, doctors may not have time to look at every clinical condition, so, by cooperating, they can exchange personalized information and find the most efficient solution. In the third scenario doctors recommend websites to their patients so as to educate them so they can filter the information gained from their web searches.

---

[191]   Miriam McMullan, "Patients using the Internet to obtain health information: How this affects the patient–health professional relationship," *Patient Education and Counselling* 63, (2006): 24–28.

Conclusions

As we have seen, medicine (and philosophy of medicine), can create different world views, with different foundations and different metaphysical presuppositions. This was clarified in our analysis by the presentation of the two main forms of medical reasoning, the biomedical or objective and the humanistic or subjective. The biomedical model is based on a materialistic and mechanistic view of the body; consequently, the patient is conceived of as an entity, which is a collection of parts with an appropriate function; when this appropriate function is interrupted, we have a manifestation of disease. Doctors seek to substantiate knowledge which will be valid in every social or cultural context and will not be distorted by the possible biased personal values of the patient. The ultimate aim is to achieve patient safety and reduce errors in medical praxis. There are two main methods of that value-free medical reasoning: reasoning based on statistics and evidence-based medicine. Bayesian statistics are used for the prediction of a future event; therefore, when a clinical trial is being held it can be terminated earlier so less patients are exposed to a possibly ineffective or harmful therapy, or we can evaluate the efficacy of one drug. Frequentist statistics, on the other hand, are used for the comparison of two patient groups. In short, a null hypothesis and an alternative hypothesis is made; the first suggests that there will not be a significant statistical difference between the two groups and the second is that there will be. If the calculations lead to the rejection of the null hypothesis, the group that received the most beneficial treatment will be second group. Evidence-based medicine aims at the reduction of the dependence on the intuition of the doctor and the non-systematic clinical experience. Doctors should have (or obtain) the capacity of bibliographical research in an effective way and the application of tools that critically evaluate clinical research. In general, it is a systematic application of rules and directions that a doctor has to follow in medical praxis: how to reject or apply a proposed protocol, by what criteria, etc. It is summarized as "the conscientious, explicit, and judicious use of current best evidence in making decisions about the care of individual patients."[192] The subjective or humanistic model of reasoning is not based on quantified methods—i.e., mathematical or statistical models. It focuses on the meaning of the illness attributed by the patients and their subjective ex-

---

[192]   D. L. Sackett, W. M. Rosenberg, J. A. Gray, R. B. Haynes, and W. S. Richardson, "Evidence-Based Medicine: What it Is and What it Isn't," *British Medical Journal*, no. 312 (1996): 71–72.

perience. It is based on a holism that tries to involve the interaction of the patient with his family, society, and healthcare practitioners. The patient is a particularity with a subjective experience of pain, despair, and incapability of performing vital functions, such as difficulties in breathing. Furthermore, he is an entity with existential or religious concerns. The illness therefore is not simply a "malfunction of the body", a disorder in the body chemistry, or the presence of a pathogen in a biological system, but rather a transformation of personal experience. When the first-person experience is not taken into account, there could be a reduction in the understanding of how a therapeutic intervention is experienced, by which kind of emotions it is accompanied, or how it is inscribed in memory. Given that both disease and the respective therapeutic methods can vitally change the life of the patient, it needs to be understood how these events alter the patient's self-understanding in ways that possibly are beyond "quantification" and can standardize a "quality of life". Lastly, we seek to explore the doctor-patient relationship, with emphasis on the information age. We first refer to classical model of conceptualization like those proposed by Szasz and Hollender as well as Emanuel and Emmauel, and proceed then to the new status that the digitally engaged patient adopts through his interaction with cyber environments, and how this affects both the status and his relationship with the physicians.

Chapter 5:
The Impact of Big Data on Medicine

Introduction

Big Data generated in the domain of health and biological sciences has progressively revolutionized and changed our biomedical approach. We speak more and more about integrative biology and personalized medicine Bioinformatics and biostatistics provide powerful tools for management and analysis of various data such as biomarkers, the expenses of the health care system, patients' follow-up, environmental factors, everyday habits, etc. Additionally, the evolution of systems biology and the "omic" technologies (genomics, proteomics, metabolomics...) have contributed to the creation of preventive and predictive formulas of certain diseases.

Our aim is, on the one hand, to present the methods of data analysis and knowledge acquisition: data mining, machine learning, and deep learning, and on the other hand to reflect upon their efficacy and limits. Additionally, we focus our attention on the role of internet 2.0 in medical practice, presenting its advantages and disadvantages. After a historical approach to the various models of categorization of disease (taxonomy) and their particular contribution to our current methodologies, we refer to the need for categorization of disease on a molecular basis. Furthermore, we uncover epistemological and philosophical questions deeply linked to Big Data. First, what are the limits of Big Data and randomized control trials and is there a need for observational studies? Second, we seek to explore what happens with the empiricism that Big Data brought, claiming that correlation is enough. Consequently, we compare the classical hypothetico-deductive medical reasoning with abductive reasoning, as proposed by Alexander Gungov in his *Patient Safety: The Relevance of Logic in Medical Care*. Third, since Big Data is generated through various scientific fields, we approach their interdisciplinarity through Anne-Françoise Schmid's and M. Mambrini-Doudet's *Epistemologie Generique*. We then focus on Emmanuel Levinas's primacy of ethics and Derrida's ethics of the un-decisional in comparison to some of the basic assumptions of this thesis, such as glaring. Finally, we approach the definition of disease through the prism of the debate between naturalism and normativism.

5.1 Omic technologies

The explosion of omic technologies goes in parallel with (bio)informatics, as well as a fundamental theory of discrete fields contributing to the birth of these extraordinary advances. The grounding theory before 1950 could be summarized as follows: In the 1930s, Graph Theory was the tool proposed in mathematics for network analysis. In the 1940sand 1950s, focused programs promoted the idea of the applied and general purpose of computers, e.g., Manchester Mark 1, EDSAC, etc. Alan Turing's assumption that physical and mathematical laws can be applied in biological systems was popular in the 1950s (although this can be traced back to Charles Darwin under the influence of Thomas Robert Malthus' demographics). Finally, the *General Systems Theory* of Ludwig Von Bertalanffy called for an interdisciplinary approach among sciences in which exact formulas are generalized to common systems between the various scientific domains.[193]

Evolution in patient care and preventive medicine has been recorded after the emergence of the human genome project and the studies of the microbiome. As presented in *Toward Precision Medicine: Building a Knowledge Network for Biomedical Research and a New Taxonomy of Disease* (2011), high cholesterol is correlated with the onset of coronary disease. One among 500 individuals is heterozygous for a non-functional variant of the low-density-lipoprotein-receptor gene. The regulation of everyday habits is not sufficient for the reduction of probabilities concerning an early onset. Following the above facts, the recognition of patients with this type of genome and the quick administration of statins is recommended.[194] Mutations in BRCA1 and BRCA2 tumor suppressors predispose for ovarian and mammary cancer[195]; the distribution among patients

---

[193]   A detailed overview, both of the history of the rise of omics data and the methods of their analysis and the associated problems, is found in the work of C. Manzoni, D. Kia, J. Vandrovcova, J. Hardy, N. Wood, P. Lewis, & R. Ferrari, "Genome, transcriptome and proteome: the rise of omics data and their integration in biomedical sciences," Briefings in Bioinformatics, no. 19 (2016): 286–302.

[194]   R Huijgen,. M.N. Vissers, J.C. Defesche, P.J. Lansberg, J.J. Kastelein, and B.A. Hutten, "Familial hypercholesterolemia: Current treatment and advances in management," *Expert Rev.Cardiovasc.* no.6 (2008): 567–81.

[195]   M.C King, J.H. Marks, J.B. Mandell, and the New York Breast Cancer Study Group, "Breast and ovarian cancer risks due to inherited mutations in BRCA1 and BRCA2," *Science*, no. 302 (2003): 643–46.

in the US is estimated at 0.06% for the former and 0.4% for the latter[196]. The risk can be eliminated by regular cancer screening and prophylactic breast and ovary removal surgeries.[197] Stomach ulcers seem to be linked nowadays with the bacterium *helicobacter pylori*. Successful treatment can cure not only the ulcers but also reduce the possibility of stomach cancer, which is closely connected to the ulcers[198]. MODY (Maturity Onset of Diabetes of the Young) is approached today as having a relation with specific genetic variants that affect pancreatic beta cell function[199].

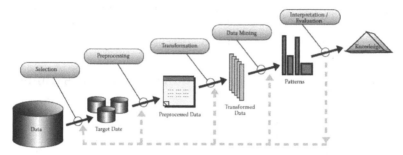

Figure 3. KDD process © copyright : Fayyad, U., Piatetsky-Shapiro, G., & Smyth, P. (1996). From Data Mining to Knowledge Discovery in Databases. *AI Magazine, 17*(3), 37. https://doi.org/10.1609/aimag.v17i3. 1230

5.2 From Three Vs to Five Vs—Characterization of Big Data

In the beginning, Big Data was characterized under a scheme of three Vs (volume, velocity, and variety); in time, two new complementary characteristics were added (value, and veracity or validity), for their economic

196   K.E.Malone, J.R. Daling, D.R. Doody, L. Hsu, L. Bernstein, R.J. Coates, P.A. March-banks, M.S.Simon, J.A. McDonald, S.A. Norman, B.L. Strom, R.T. Burkman, G. Ursin, D. Deapen, L.K.Weiss, S. Folger, J.J. Madeoy, D.M. Friedrichsen, N.M. Suter, M.C. Humphrey, R. Spirtas,and E.A. Ostrander, "Prevalence and predictors of BRCA1 and BRCA2 mutations in apopulation-based study of breast cancer in white and black American women ages 35 to 64 years," *Cancer Res*, no. 66 (2006):8297–308.

197   D.H Roukos, and E. Briasoulis, "Individualized preventive and therapeutic management of hereditary breast ovarian cancer syndrome," *Nat. Clin. Pract. Oncol*, no.4 (2001): 578–90.

198   J.C. Atherton. *The pathogenesis of Helicobacter pylori-induced gastro-duodenal diseases. Annual Review of Pathology*, no. 1 (2006): 63–96.

199   S.S Fajans, G.I. Bell, K.S. Polonsky, "Molecular mechanisms and clinical pathophysiology of maturity-onset diabetes of the young," *New England. Journal of medicine*, no. 345 (2001): 971–80.

and ethical dimensions could be encapsulated: a) volume, the basic reason behind the term "Big", referring to the quantity of information, of a very big volume, to be acquired, stored, treated, analyzed, and transmitted by standard tools; b) velocity, which describes the dynamic aspect of Big Data in relation with time, the difficulty of the actualization and analysis; the data are treated in real time or quasi-real time (streaming); c) variety, linked with the heterogeneity of formats, types, and quality of information; d) value, a complementary characteristic which refers to the potentiality of data more particularly in economic terms; and e) veracity or validity, a complementary characteristic which lies in the quality of data and the ethical problems inherent to its use[200].

5.3 How New Knowledge is Acquired from Data Mining

Fayaad et al. (1996)[201] summarize knowledge acquisition in nine steps; this is the so-called KDD process:

1st step: To understand the domain of application and if there should be some prior knowledge

2nd step: To create a target data set (focus on sets of variables or data samples)

3rd step: Data cleaning and processing (mainly noise reduction and management of missing data)

4th step: Data reduction and projection, e.g., dimensionality reduction

5th step: Matching the goals of step 1 with a particular data mining method: regression, clustering, etc.

6th step: Exploratory analysis and modeling and hypothesis selection (e.g., models of categorical data, models of vectors)

7th step: Data mining in which we search for patterns of interest in a particular representational form or sets of this kind of representations (trees, regression, clustering)

8th step: Interpretation and visualization of mined patterns

9th step: How we act upon the discovered knowledge, e.g., by making a direct use of knowledge, by incorporating it in another

---

[200]   Cf. B.Espinasse, P.Bellot, "Introduction au Big Data Opportunités, stockage et analyse des mégadonnées," *Technologies De L'information | Technologies Logicielles Architectures Des Systèmes* (2001).

[201]   Fayyad, Usama, Gregory Piatetsky-Shapiro, and Padhraic Smyth, "From Data Mining to Knowledge Discovery in Databases," *AI Magazine*, no. 17 (1996): 37

system, by documentation, or, finally, by a resolution of potential conflicts with regard to previous knowledge.

The methods of algorithmic analysis of big data can be divided in three broad categories:

Non-supervised methods: They are purely exploratory; they permit us to organize and summarize the available information. We could distinguish: a) factor analysis (principal component analysis, exploratory factor analysis), b) partition (k-means) and hierarchy (ascending hierarchy classification), c) association (a-priori association), and d) correlation analysis.[202]

Supervised methods: They permit us to explain a variable with the help of other variables. Secondly, since the value of this variable of interest is unknown, they permit us to predict this value, naturally with an error of prediction. We speak about supervised methods if the attribute of a variable is quantitative or binary (logistic regression, decision trees, neuron networks, Bayesian networks, discrimination analysis). Otherwise, we speak generally about regressions, e.g., for explanation or prediction of quantitative variables (linear regression), or for calculus (Poisson regression, tree of Poisson, etc.)[203]

Semi-Supervised: the balancing of performance and precision by the use of small sets of labeled or annotated data in parallel with a much larger unlabeled data collection.[204]

Specific mathematical models are used in the following cases:

Clustering: is used in phylogenetic analysis; also we can redefine the disease according to physiopathological criteria and achieve more specified treatments. Microarray data analysis permitted the approach of different types of lymphoma among diagnosed patients by making a com-

---

[202]   Cf. Emmanuel Chazard, "Réutilisation et fouille de données massives de santé produites en routine au cours du soin" (HdR diss.,LilleUniversité, 2016).

[203]   Ibid.

[204]   Cf. Ivo Dinov, "Methodological challenges and analytic opportunities for modeling and interpreting Big Healthcare Data," *GigaSience*, no.5 (2001).

parison of the clusters' similarly expressed genes and whether or not they responded to the current therapy.[205]

Linear Regression: Longitudinal analysis of data. Reed et al. (2013)[206] found that implementing an Electronic Health Record in patients suffering from diabetes mellitus had a moderate effect in the reduction in ED visits and hospitalizations and no effect on office visit rates. After a large-scale hypertension program in northern California, they had significant control in comparison with state and national control rates.[207] Yuasa et al. (2011)[208] researched the correlation between the initial tumor sizes of patients treated with targeted agents and found that only the initial tumor size is correlated with the reduction rate in individual tumors.

Logistic regression: De Vries et al. (2010)[209] explored the mortality of iatrogenic diseases outside the operation room.[210] The majority of the medical emergencies during flights were associated with respiratory and gastro-intestinal symptoms.

Epigenetics: Fu et al. (2010) developed methods of Bayesian inference on Big Data epigenetics in order to study the transmission of DNA methylation during cellular multiplication.[211]

Machine learning: Machine learning concerns the acquisition of data and the elaboration of algorithms capable of determining the common points between two populations by the use of statistical methods.

[205]   Alizadeh, MB Eisen, RE Davis, C Ma, IS, Lossos, A. Rosenwald , et al, "Distinct types of diffuse large B-cell lymphoma identified by gene expression profiling," *Nature* , no.11 (2000): 403–503.

[206]   M.ReeJ.Huang , R.Brand , I.Graetz , R.Neugebauer , B.Fireman , et al., "Implementation of an outpatient electronic health record and emergency department visits, hospitalizations, and office visits among patients with diabetes," *JAMA, no.* 310 (2013): 1060–65.

[207]   Jaffe MG, Lee GA, Young JD, Sidney S, Go AS, "Improved blood pressure control associated with a large-scale hypertension program," *JAMA*, no. 310 (2016): 699–705.

[208]   T. Yuasa, S. Urakami, S. Yamamoto, J Yonese, K. Nakano, M. Kodaira, et al., "Tumor size is a potential predictor of response to tyrosine kinase inhibitors in renal cell cancer," *Urology*, no. 77 (2001): 831–35.

[209]   EN De Vries, HA Prins RM Crolla, AJ den Outer, G van Andel, SH van Helde, et al, "Effect of a comprehensive surgical safety system on patient outcomes," *N Engl J Med*, no. 363 (2010): 1928–37

[210]   DC Peterson, C Martin-Gill, FX Guyette, AZ Tobias, CE McCarthy, ST Harrington, et al., "Outcomes of medical emergencies on commercial airline flights," *N Engl J Med*, no. 368 (2011): 2075–83.

[211]   AQ Fu, DP Genereux, R Stoger, CD Laird, M Stephens, "Statistical inference of transmission fidelity of DNA methylation patterns over somatic cell divisions in mammals," Ann Appl Stat, no. 4 (2010): 871–92.

The exploitation of data created by machine learning permits us to treat a great number of variables and registries.[212]

Deep learning: Deep learning is based on the concept of neuron networks. These methods are based on probabilistic methods of a Bayesian type already used, for example, in the protocols of clinical research for enhancing strength.[213]

Algorithmic analyses of 2032 cases were compared with a study of a group of 21 experts after deep learning performed in a bank of images. The obtained results were comparable in terms of specificity and sensibility, and in the majority of cases were better for the deep learning algorithm. In conclusion, the prospects of the use of this algorithm, coupled with the use of smart phones, for collecting the images of skin abnormalities, proposes a significant extension in the prevention of dermatological cancers.[214]

Google flu trends was an attempt to predict the spread of flu. The results of a study realized in eight countries of South America between 2012 and 2014 were not completely audited. They were better in Mexico and the authors suggest that the correlation is higher in countries with a subtropical climate. It is also an attempt to use data from social networks and not only from health-related databases[215].

A deep learning algorithm developed by Google in collaboration with the University of Texas at Austin was used for detection of retinal disease in patients suffering from diabetes mellitus. From a base of 128,175 images, two samples of 9963 and 1748 were used for validation. The specificity of the second test was 96.2% and the sensibility, 93.9%, comparable with the results of seven specialists who also interpreted the images. The authors reveal the present limits of the systems such as the difficulty of the algorithm in the analysis of images with different mate-

---

[212] Jean Patrick Lajochere, "Role of Big Data in evolution of the medical practice," Bull. Acad. NatleMéd., séance du 6 février 2018

[213] Jean Patrick Lajochere, "Role of Big Data in evolution of the medical practice" Bull. Acad. Natle Méd., séance du février 6, 2018.

[214] A Esteva, B Kuprel, R Novoa, J Ko, S Swetter, H Blau,S Thrun, "Dermatologist-level classification of skin cancer with deep neural networks," Nature, no. 542 (2017): 115–18.

[215] Simon Pollett, W. John Boscardin, Eduardo Azziz-Baumgartner, Yeny O. Tinoco, Giselle Soto, Candice Romero, Jen Kok, Matthew Biggerstaff, Cecile Viboud, George W. Rutherford, "Evaluating Google Flu Trends in Latin America: Important Lessons for the Next Phase of Digital Disease Detection, *Clinical Infectious Diseases,* no. 64 (2017): 34–41.

rial and the superiority of the specialists who were capable of detecting lesions, which the program was unable to detect.[216]

5.4 The Role of the Internet (Web 2.0)

The internet, and more specifically web 2.0 (user-generated content and the growth of social media), can be a beneficial tool both for physicians and patients. For the former it permits easier access to bibliography and medical databases. Furthermore, through the establishment of various medical communities, a broader exchange of medical information can be achieved almost in real time or quasi-real time, consequently achieving more specialized treatments and protocols, encapsulating a more evidence-based medical approach. Concerning the patients, they may benefit from telemedical practices especially if they live in remote places; those with cases of chronic diseases can participate in online support groups, share common experiences, and possibly adopt a more active role in the way they perceive their disease. Furthermore, some surveys reveal a reduction of suffering and pain in people participating in this kind of group. We can focus a bit more on the notion of the patient's active role if we also account for the phenomenon of health seekers (individuals accessing sites related to diseases, medical treatments, health care services, etc.). This phenomenon has a bifid character as to its advantages and major disadvantages.[217] We will briefly enumerate some of them. The advantages are: a) the patient becomes aware of his disease and consequently can adopt the character of a well-informed patient, so he is more likely to comply with prescribed medical treatments, have a sense of control over the disease, or take actions that he may have not taken otherwise; b) the clinical time may be used more efficiently (presuming that the patient has access to reliable information); thus information exchange between doctor and patient can be more focused on treatment options and decision-making, and c) after the visit, the information may be augmented and patients may be more satisfied or comfortable with a proposed treatment, which can be described as a priming effect. The disadvantages are: a) the reliability, or the information obtained may be

---

[216]   Cf.V Gulshan . et al., "Development and validation of a deep learning algorithm for detection of diabetic retinopathy in retinal fundus photographs," *JAMA* (2016).

[217]   Hedy S. Wald, Catherine E. Dube, David C. Anthony, "Untangling the Web: The impact of Internet use on health care and the physician–patient relationship," *Patient Education and Counseling*, no. 63 (2006): 24–28.

misleading or misinterpreted,[218] which may result in requesting inappropriate interventions or examinations, tests, and unnecessary visits,[219] or
may have an effect of over-anxiety that may lead to morbidity and even
mortality;[220] b) the way socioeconomic disparities affect the access to
information (income, age, and familiarity with new technologies); and c)
issues of liability such as cases in which the patients find the standards of
provided care inferior to the way presented on the web.[221]

---

[218]   We will refer at least to three studies targeted to the cases of misleading information and
liability: The first is related to Youtube and medical information about orthodontics. In a
scan of 5140 results, the majority of videos uploaded were by patients and not by a specialist; these videos were also the most popular. The content of the videos as well as the
quality of the information met low standards of quality, with a vague presentation of the
profession of the orthodontist. The majority of the contributions by regular orthodontists
were advertising, something with a negative effect on the Youtube users, who favored
the videos uploaded by patients. (Michael Knosel, Klaus Jung, "Information Value and
bias of videos related to orthodontics screened on a video-sharing Website," *Angle Orthod*, no. 81 (2011): 532–39.) The second study concerns Twitter and the sharing of information on the use of antibiotics. The study confirmed that Twitter is a space in which
medical information and advice is shared informally. The diffusion of information mainly through networks and retweets contains both valid and invalid information. Positive
behaviors can be adopted and real-time medical data can be extracted. The study concludes with the importance of the understanding of the role and popularity of the social
media by healthcare professionals and the nature of the health-related information shared
there. (D. Scanfeld, V. Scanfeld , E. Larson, "Dissemination of health information
through social networks: Twitter and antibiotics," *Am J Infect Control* , no. 38 (2010):
182–88.) The last one unveils the role of Wikipedia as a source of drug information. We
cite the findings as presented: Wikipedia was able to answer significantly fewer drug information questions (40.0%) compared with MDR (82.5%; $p < 0.001$). Wikipedia performed poorly regarding information on dosing, with a score of 0% versus the MDR
score of 90%. Answers found in Wikipedia were 76% complete, while MDR provided
answers that were 95.5% complete; overall, Wikipedia answers were less complete than
those in Medscape ($p < 0.001$). No factual errors were found in Wikipedia, whereas 4 answers in Medscape conflicted with the answer key; errors of omission were higher in
Wikipedia (n = 48) than in MDR (n = 14). There was a marked improvement in Wikipedia over time, as current entries were superior to those 90 days prior ($p = 0.024$). The
study concludes that it had weaker results than the compared database and therefore is
not authoritative and can be used only as supplementary by consumers for their information. K. Clauson, H. Polen, M. Kamel Boulos, J. Dzenogiannis, "Scope, completeness, and accuracy of drug information in Wikipedia," Ann Pharmakometer, no. 42
(2008): 1814–21.
[219]   E. Murray, B. Lo, F Pollack, K. Donelan, J. Catania, M. White, K Zapert, R Turner,
"The impact of health information on the internet on the physician–patient relationship," *Arch Intern Med*, no. 163 (2003): 1727–34.
[220]   SD Weisbord, JB Soule, PL Kimmel, "Poison on line—acute renal failure caused by
oil of wormwood purchased through the Internet," *NEJM*, no.72. (1997): 825–7.
[221]   Hedy S. Wald, Catherine E. Dube, David C. Anthony, "Untangling the Web—The
impact of Internet use on health care and the physician–patient relationship," *Patient
Education and Counseling*, no. 63 (2006): 24–28

5.5 A Brief History of Taxonomy

Thomas Sydenham pioneered a view, in his *Medical Practice* (1666), by proclaiming that we should categorize diseases by their precise and determinate species, like the botanists had done in their work on plants.[222] In the history of scientific classification of disease we could also highlight the attempt of Carolus Linnaeus. In his *Genera Morborum* (1763), he classified diseases in three broad categories, exanthematic (fever and skin eruptions), phlogistic (fever, heavy pulse, topical pain), and dolorous (pain).[223] In the *Dictionary of Medical Sciences, From the Society of Physicians and Surgeons, Edition of Panchoucke*, we find the definition of nosography as the science describing diseases. It is composed of the Greek *nosos* (disease) and *grafo* (describe). Furthermore, having achieved the denomination of nosology, it can attain more proper signification used for titling works devoted principally to the descriptive part of diseases.[224] Philippe Pinel, in his *Philosophical Nosography or the Applied Method in Medical Analysis* (1862), proposes that diseases should not be considered as a constantly flexible field, an incoherent assemblage of affections, contributing to an endless debate over remedies, but as the sum of characteristic symptoms with successive periods according to a natural tendency, which is in most cases favorable but sometimes leads to disasters. Claude Bernard, in his *Introduction to the Study of Experimental Medicine* (1865), underlines the experimental character of the classification of diseases, claiming that a physician does not acquire knowledge of a disease if he does not act rationally and experimentally towards it, in the same way that a zoologist does not know the animals and instead explains and regulates the phenomenon of life.[225] Nowadays, the International Classification of Diseases (ICD, currently ICD 11), published and revised by the World Health Organization (WHO), is considered the most usual protocol of disease categorization.[226]

---

[222] Médecine pratique de Sydenham. Avec des notes. Ouvrage traduit en français sur la dernière ed. Anglaise par M.A.F. Jault Paris 1784 (préface des observations, 1666). Préface de l'auteur.

[223] National Research Council. *Toward Precision Medicine: Building a Knowledge Network for Biomedical Research and a New Taxonomy of Disease* (Washington, DC: The National Academies Press,2011),12.

[224] *Dictionnaire des sciences médicales, par une société de médecins et de chirurgiens, édition* de Panchoucke, Paris, 1819, article "Nosographie".

[225] Claude Bernard, *Introduction à la médecine expérimentale, considérations expérimentales spéciales aux êtres vivants* (Paris : Livre de poche, 1988), 319–320.

[226] National Research Council, *Toward Precision Medicine: Building a Knowledge Network for Biomedical Research and a New Taxonomy of Disease* 2011, 12.

5.6 The Need for the Categorization of Disease on a Molecular Basis

The Committee on A Framework for Developing a New Taxonomy of Disease. Board on Life Sciences, Division on Earth and Life Studies, National Research Council in the US have called for a new categorization of disease on a molecular basis after the tremendous changes in omic technologies. In order for this project to be realized, a new knowledge network of disease has to be developed. Through this network, an information commons which is individual-centric and combines the knowledge of biology will encapsulate the causal influence and the mechanisms of pathogenesis involved in an individual's health. By hypothesizing new intra-layer cluster analysis, researchers could determine new diseases or subtypes of diseases that are clinically relevant. The purpose of these two projects (an information commons and a knowledge network) is summarized in three directions briefly delineated below: a) the creation of a dynamic and flexible system which informs the classification of disease; b) a new grounding of tailor-made clinical praxis (diagnosis, treatment, and decision-making); and c) a system for basic discovery. A Geographic Information System (GIS)-type structure is proposed for organizing the information commons. Practically, it is a method of layering in which the bottom layer defines the organization of the overlays. The particularity of the medical information commons lies in the fact that it is distinct from the GIS in which the layering has as its foundational geographical position. The data in each of the higher layers overlay on the patient layer in complex ways (e.g., patients with similar microbiomes and symptoms may have very different genome sequences).[227]

5.7 The Limits of Big Data and Randomized Control Trials (RCTs)

One of the first and crucial limitations of Big Data in health and biology is faced when we pass from Big Data to smart data, meaning the data which can be used in real time and effectively for a particular case (prevention, prognosis, diagnosis, and therapeutics).[228] Two also important

---

[227] Ibid., 17.
[228] GW Ewing, "The limitations of big data in healthcare," *MOJ Proteomics Bioinform,* no. 5 (2017): 40–43.

limitations arising from the nature of statistical analysis are the curse of dimensionality and missing values. The first was introduced by Richard Bellman in the 1950s and revealed the optimization problem in high-dimensional datasets. The method of data handling that proposes to remove cases with missing values or perform a complete-case analysis is efficient only if the missing values are independent of both observed and unobserved data. This fact is not usual in praxis, so a complete case analysis could bias the conclusion. Finally, by reducing the number of data points available, a complete case analysis seems to be extremely inefficient.[229] Beyond these problems revolving around statistical analysis, when it turns to the application of Big Data in models explaining biological functions (biomarker-type tests), many questions can arise concerning the in vivo regulation of hormone levels, the detection of pathological correlations, or the way the autonomic nervous system and organs are regulated by the brain. Therefore, the reliability and the meta-theoretical background of these methods is under reconsideration: "Is the biomarker the cause or the consequence of a pathological condition? Is there a relation between the biomarker and the genotype, the phenotype or neither?"[230]

Randomized control trials (RTCs) are considered to be the gold standard for medical research. Cartwright and Deaton call for a rethinking, not a total critique, of their efficacy and their limits in particular cases, and we will briefly refer to some of them.[231] The first is that prior knowledge is needed for implementing this or that protocol, or analyzing its results. This knowledge may come from observational studies, which will be integrated with other knowledge like the practical wisdom of policymakers. Prior knowledge could also be needed in cases like the analysis of the human genome. Out of billions of base pairs, only some of them, or even one of them, might be important, and if these particular bases are found to be unbalanced, then the results of a trial can be randomly confounded and untrue. Consequently, we should calculate the proper length of the bases used, so that the above errors can be avoided. Although RTCs can minimize bias and handle the issues of confounding,

[229]   C Lee, H Yoon, "Medical big data: promise and challenges," Kidney Research and Clinical Practice, no. 36 (2017): 3–11.

[230]   Ibid.

[231]   For more see: August Deaton, "Instruments, Randomization and Learning about Development," Journal of Economic Literature, no. 48 (2010): 424–455, Cartwrigh Nancy, "Are RCTs the Gold Standard," iosocieties, no. 2 (2008): 11–20., Cartwright, Nancy, "What Are Randomised Controlled Trials Good For?," Philosophical Studies, no. 147 (2010): 59–70.

sometimes they are far from having a generalizing character. They are conducted under almost ideal conditions, following very strict protocols of patient selection; additionally, they cannot always be performed due to practical and ethical reasons.

5.8 Data-Driven/Hypothesis-Driven/Hypothetico-Deductive Medical Reasoning in Comparison with Alexander Gungov's Interpretation of Abductive Method in *Patient Safety: The Relevance of Logic in Medical Care*

Is the Big Data era accompanied by the fourth paradigmatic change in science—data-intensive, exploratory, and dependent on data mining methods— as Jim Gray proclaims?[232] Can we really speak of the end of theory and a new emerging empiricism, following the influential article by Chris Anderson,[233] former editor-in-chief of *Wired* magazine? According to Anderson, petabytes can lead us to claim that correlation is enough; data can be analyzed without making any hypotheses. The algorithms are more performative than science for producing patterns. Causation is passed by correlation, and science does not demand necessarily coherent modeling, unification of theories, and explanatory methods. Rob Kitchin[234] summarizes this new dominant empiricist approach in four points: a) Big Data covers a full domain by providing concrete resolutions; b) a priori theory, modeling, and hypotheses are not essential; c) the agnostic nature of data analytics can speak for itself and, overcoming inherent human bias, can lead to meaningful and truthful patterns and associations; and d) the knowledge of a specific domain is not needed; in science meaning transcends context, and consequently, anyone adept at statistics can be an interpreter. John Symons and Ramon Alvarado[235] contend that plenty of authors—on the one hand—understand the important role Big Data plays in the resolution of problems not easily

[232]   Cf. Hey, Anthony J. G, Stewart Tansley, Kristin Michele Tolle, *The Fourth Paradigm* (Redmond, Wash.: Microsoft Research, 2009).
[233]   Chris Anderson, "The end of theory: The data deluge makes the scientific method obsolete," *Wired*, June 23, 2008, http://www.wired.com/science/discoveries/magazine/16-07/pb_theory, last accessed, December 25, 2020.
[234]   Rob Kitchin, "Big Data, New Epistemologies and Paradigm Shifts," *Big Data & Society*, (April, 2014).
[235]   Cf. Symons, John, and Ramón Alvarado, "Can We Trust Big Data? Applying Philosophy of Science to Software," Big Data & Society, no. 3 (2016).

reached before,[236] but—on the other—criticize this statistical empiricism concerning its epistemological basis. The first concerns the new knowledge acquired from data mining. Lazer et al.[237] call us to rethink the reliability of data and science that are not an outcome of the use of scientific instruments. The other major problem is if Big Data analysis is linked with an epistemic opacity.[238] A process, according to Humphrey, is epistemically opaque, relative to a cognitive agent X at time t, if X does not know at t all of the epistemically relevant elements of the process. Epistemic opacity is reinforced if we also consider the fact that algorithmic errors can occur; there are different proposed methods such as severe testing.[239] The authors call for a new conception in the philosophy of statistics, in which the reliability of a hypothesis is relevant to the fact that it has been falsified by a test. In this method, the selection of a hypothesis is by virtue of the extent of error-detecting tests. The last one concerns the complexity of Big Data analysis (distribution of errors, coding, testing, and the management of black boxes).

This kind of almost agonistic empiricism brings forth the need for an approach in medical practice that combines the idea of the patient's safety under the spectrum of logic, as posed by Gungov, the interdisciplinarity between sciences and science-philosophy/science-ethics in a *generic* conception of epistemology, as Anne- Françoise Schmid and Muriel Mambrini-Doudet thoroughly analyze, and finally, returning to our basic assumptions, the rethinking of Emmanuel Levinas and his uncertainty of knowing as positivity and Jacques Derrida in his ethics of the un-decisional in comparison with the notion of performativity of action, and, of course, trace and real-semblance. Gungov not only gives a detailed analysis of the various fallacies occurring in diagnostics and therapeutics and proposes their respective resolution (a combination of abductive reasoning mainly after Charles Sanders Peirce, speculative thinking, and Giambattista Vico's idea of *verum factum*), but he also reveals the

---

[236]   A. Barberousse, S. Franceschelli, C. Imbert, "Computer simulations as experiments," Synthese, no. 169 (2009): 557–574, Barberousse A., Vorms M, "About the Empirical Warrants of Computer-Based Scientific Knowledge," Synthese, Springer Verlag (Germany), no. 191 (2014): 3595-620.

[237]   Lazer D., Kennedy R., King G., et al., "The parable of Google Flu: Traps in big data analysis," Science, no. 334 (2016):434.

[238]   P. Humphrey, "The philosophical novelty of computer simulation methods," Synthese, no. 169 (2008): 615–626.

[239]   Cf. DG. Mayo and A. Spanos, Error and Inference: Recent Exchanges on Experimental Reasoning, Reliability, and the Objectivity and Rationality of Science (New York, NY: Cambridge University Press, 2010).

enigmatic character of health (as Hans-Georg Gadamer claims) and, finally, does not abandon the political and ethical necessity over the extreme quantification of the patient and the danger of becoming a "statistical unit", as well as the impossibility and incapacity of automatic statistical reasoning. Gungov, as we said above, proposes pragmatic abductive medical reasoning over the deductive and inductive. First, the individual (result) is inferred from the universal (rule) through the particularity (the case). So, if we consider this regarding clinical praxis, the physician starts from the already registered information (articles, medical books, etc.) as reflecting the universal (rule), and essentially has to end at some results which may be verified or falsified. Induction from the other is directed from the individual reasoning (result) to the universal rule, thus ending up only with probable results, which may be either true or false after testing. Abductive reasoning is from the other context; it relies on experience as well as decision strategy. Heuristic hypotheses are justified rationally by the present data.[240] Consequently, if we consider Big Data, when a physician has to pass to smart data (from a patient to this patient), he can dynamically start from the sign of a disease (consequences) and look for the reasons. Observations which may contain laboratory results, clinical results after examination, and even smart data from an algorithm, e.g. a data-mined image of a cancer, are in continuous reconsideration and reevaluation based on differential diagnosis; the method of exclusion and disjunctive syllogism and their truthfulness are further tested by the theories of coherence and correspondence.[241] This "doing after thinking" of course demands the "exploitation" of the patient (individuality) as the source of the medical data (signs, symptoms, etc.), but can pass beyond what is contained in the universal.

To continue our analysis, not only Big Data, but also new advancements in biotechnology, like GMOs (salmon) and new fields of research like those on cancer, Alzheimer's disease, and climate change can give us the essence of how common (interdisciplinary) objects become scientific objects, according to Schmid and Mambrini-Doudet.[242] This object is an integrative object which has at least three characteristics: "it is an object a) that acts in relation with the object, to pose it better, complexity is not sufficient to describe the contemporary objects. b)

---

[240]   Alexander Gungov, *Patient Safety: The Relevance Of Logic In Medical Care* (Sttugard: ibidem Press,2018), 60.

[241]   Ibid., 97.

[242]   Anne-Françoise Schmid and Muriel Mambrini-Doudet, *Épistémologie Générique* (Paris: kime, 2019), 70.

The integrative object invites a dynamic of the knowledge, of exchanging flux between heterogeneous knowing, which do not have a definitive end. c) It is not synthesizable."[243] In another passage they describe the notion of the data-given as the motor engine of their research: "the notion of the fact may be abandoned gradually and give its place to the data-given ... the data- given is not yet a correlate of a theory. The data-given gives the ordering of the magnitude, it is generic, multiplied, disposable, there is no order of magnitude assigned to it".[244]

Following Maria Dimitrova,[245] the moral subject, according to Levinas,[246] constitutes itself not from an action and a reaction, but by the speech and conversation. A real conversation is both instructive and apologetic. It presupposes greeting, attention, and respect for the Other. The relation **one-for-the-Other** is the primordial rationality. Justice is a principle imposed from beyond being and is a mode of behavior if it is based on the authenticity of the Other. The dramatic character of the human is an immediate and prior reference to the language where the said betrays the saying. The philosophy of the 20th century focuses its attention on language and speech. The pre-logical orientation to the Other is that non-intentional consciousness that Levinas describes. The **me** always reaches the third one, the third one is the Other but is qualified by an entity on a territoriality. As God commanded, **thou shall not** and men responded to his call, this command does not derive from **you can**, but is superior to the possible. This transcendence is for Levinas an establishment of relationship with exteriority. The **me-Other** relation, before everything else as a speaking of **Other-me**, gives meaning to the recognition of otherness. This **Other-me** relation is not constitutive for power and knowledge, but a moral relationship since the **me-Other** constantly withdraws itself from the Third.

Levinas asserts that every true word is a commandment. Before being, Logos is an appeal, the call from the Other. The approach to the Other in a conversation is equal with the breaking with any category of the Third. The Other speaking to me is a deincarnation; the discourse of a

[243]   Ibid., 71.
[244]   Ibid., 12.
[245]   Maria Dimitrova, *Sociality and Justice, Toward Social Phenomenology*, (Stuttgart: ibidem Press, 2016), 86–122.
[246]   In the paper of: kristieBall, Laura Maria Di Domenico, and Daniel Nunan., "Big Data Surveillance And The Body-Subject," *Body & Society* , no.22 (2016): 58–81. They approach ontological proximity in the context of Big Data surveillance, following Merleau-Ponty, Levinas's ethics (proximity) and Coeclekberg's digital proximity. They also emphasize the normativity and dilemmas in a local sense (proximal spaces).

conversation gives forth and triggers the meaning from one to the Other. The presence of a forwarder overcomes the anarchy of the facts and, by his (this) forwarding, determines the order, consequently the formation of a common world, shared and established by what is said. Human reason is first manifested through sociality. The relation of the one with the Other contains something divine that cannot be annihilated. We are in a manner created by the Others; the Other is still present even when absent. Our every I corresponds to the Others' appeal to me, and the very existence of the Self is already in the answer, "that is me".[247]

According to Gerard Bensussan, the ethics of the un-decisional in Derrida[248] is linked with the fact that I always have to decide about something that I do not know, between something not-known and non-sensed. Every decision is taken by the one who takes it in the temporality of this abandoning (prise-de-prise). Derrida underlines that the decision is never one. If decision already knew what was done, it would proceed until its *topos*, the possibility of already being actualized. So, it obeys the rule of always more than **one towards the two**.[249] This more than one is like **I have only one and this one is not mine**. It is a *floating* ethic in which I always **fly-sail-fly again**, ironical and an ethic close to the dominated Marrano Jewish people.[250] Later on he compares the **come** (imperative) of Derrida with the **love me** of Franz Rosenzweig. When we decide we speak a non-language, we express something unspoken; this language is the language of the Other.[251] The response of the Other is in a grammatical mode of the second person imperative which we attain, and it is only through it that we can establish an order without an order, an affirmation and a positivity without dialectics and predictive processes.[252] It can be summarized as a Messianism without Messiah.[253]

---

[247]   Maria Dimitrova, *Sociality and Justice, Toward Social Phenomenology*, (Sttugard: Ibidem Press, 2016), 86–122.

[248]   In the following papers, the notion of *Archeion* in relation with the notion of *time* in Big-Data archiving, as well as aspects of accountability, are given after a review of Jacques Derrida's *Archiving Fever, A Freudian Immersion* 1995. Daniela Agostinho, "Big Data, Time and the Archive," *symploke* 24, no. 1 (2016): 435–45, C Jeurgens, "Threats of the data-flood: An accountability perspective in the era of ubiquitous computing," in *Archives in Liquid Times*, ed. F. Smit, A. Glaudemans, & R. Jonker (Stichting Archief publicaties, 2016), 196–210.

[249]   Danielle Cohen-Levinas and Marc Crépon, *Levinas-Derrida* (Paris: Hermann.2014), 37.

[250]   Ibid.,39.

[251]   Ibid., 41.

[252]   Ibid., 44.

[253]   Ibid., 43.

Therefore, if we consider the clinical praxis from a Levinasian perspective we should keep the primacy of ethics over an uncertain decision; this uncertainty is not lack of knowledge; it has a positive essence,[254] the essence of the responsibility for the Other. Even in limiting conditions like chronic diseases, or diseases with difficulty in diagnosis, or even near-death situations, it is the Other in his fragility of his face who calls me to act in a responsible way upon him. The me-Other relationship is not an automatic one; it comes through the intermediation of the Third. If the Other in the case of Big Data is **a patient** with a not always precise figure or identity concerning his condition, if we consider raw clinical data or data from databases, when the praxis comes to "this patient" probably after acquired knowledge (data mining, machine learning, and deep learning) or after an extreme **quantification of the self** (data collected from personal wearable devices)[255], the territoriality and entity through which the Other is qualified as Third opens the relation to the exteriority. Consequently, the doctor as **being hostage to the Other** has to decide and act ethically, beyond any constitutive power or knowledge, but through speech and conversation, which demands the respect of the Other and a primordial rationality. The patient-doctor relation is "Other-me" and the doctor-patient relation is an attempt to be "me-Other". But as the Other escapes from this relationship immediately and all the time, the doctor-patient relation tends to become **me-he/she**, where **he/she** is the Third. For the real doctor, however, the **me-he/she** relation is not the goal, because the goal remains the impossible **me-Other** relation, which a good doctor strives for, and aspires to *ad infinitum*.

On the other hand, Derrida underlines the character of the decision which is always **more than one-towards the two**; our unspoken words in the second person imperative (come) expressed to the Other, attaining for his response in the temporality of that **exact time** of the decision, following the ethics of *floating*. When it turns to medical praxis, we could keep this schema for cases in which the clinical data or facts have a *bifid* character, for example, in cases in which symptoms are similar. This cannot in any case lead us in diagnosis or better differential diagno-

[254]   See the work of: Clegg, Joshua W., and Brent D. Slife, "Epistemology and the Hither Side: A Levinasian Account of Relational Knowing, *European Journal of Psychotherapy & Counselling*, no. 7 (2005): 65–76, describing Levinasian Uncertainty as positivity in their attempt to propose a Levinasian epistemology for relational knowledge in the science of psychology.

[255]   Sharon, Tamar "Self-Tracking for Health and the Quantified Self: Re-Articulating Autonomy, Solidarity, And Authenticity in an Age of Personalized Healthcare," *Philosophy & Technology*, no. 30 (2016): 93–121.

sis which presupposes a specific use of logic, and Gungov clarifies well the cases in which, for example, the symptoms are similar,[i] but still retains the very important issue of these kind of practico-ethics over a possible purely prescriptive role of a doctor violating the ethical importance of the patient, or—to put it differently—willing to impose dominance or power over the patient. In another context, ethics of *floating* could be used against the decisions of various policymakers, which can either exclude certain groups of people during the standardization of RCTs, or even stigmatization after Big Data analysis and biased interpretation of the results.

From our point of view, the relation between doctor and patient remains a one-to-one relation in relevance to a formalized context, named Dehors. The second, also important, feature is the co-existing glaring or mutual glaring which gives more place to the Levinasian Third as the one who participates in the relation not by always withdrawing from the Other, but by co-transcending the restrictive limits of a Dehors. Locality or micro-locality is also emphasized, given by the term *(o)therness*. This *(o)thereness* shares the functions of the Heideggerian (Da, as our being-in-the-world) and Hegelian (Mitte, in the chapter of Hegelian Phenomenology, Force, and Understanding, the understanding is a power that looks from the middle-mitte of the play of forces); it also refers to something as "already being there", an already existing actuality, therefore comparing it with the form of decision which Derrida describes when we have to decide we reach the *topos* of the decision (already actualized possibility). It is not dis-location; it is strictly localized; this locality does not mean that it is not affected by the micro-dynamics, since we speak about events occurring in a sublated way and eschatological exteriorizing. Reconsidering also the time of decision as the "exact" time of making the decision (prise-de-prise-abandoning), according to Derrida, we could link it with the performativity of the action. If performativity of the action is the form of evaluation that we propose, the actions performed have to be mutually glared in order to be ethical, which means to reveal the possible imposition of power and dominance in a proximal way, which means the returning trace (center from the periphery) in the one-to-one relation to be interpreted by means of a "mutual understanding" which is away from the scheme imposed by the elites or any algorithmic statistical process claiming correlation is enough: "what is to be = what is (PRIOR) to be like = to be like this" or "general signifier = real-sembling sign = sublated signified by the periphery = under a process of actualization that turns into reality".

Levinas	Relation "one-for-the-Other" primordial rationality/Primacy of Ethics/Time: Time of the Other/Eschatological-Messianic Time
Derrida	Relation "more than one-towards the two"/Ethics of *floating* (practico-ethics)/Time: Temporality of the abandoning- The "exact" time of the decision/Messianic Time without Messiah
New Proposed Model	Relation "one-to-one" in relevance with Dehors (formalized context) + glaring/Ethics of arbitrariness and performativity of the action/ Time: *(o)thereness* in relation with Dehors (Formalized context)—events in sublation/ eschatological exteriorizing—metaphysical violence of co-existing

5.9 The debate between Naturalism and Normativism

As we have seen, Big Data can provide valuable information concerning a more precise categorization of disease. Thus, we could proceed to more precise diagnostics, prognostics, and therapeutics. We have chosen to expose the various definitions of health and disease, mainly through the prism of normativism and naturalism, following Élodie Giroux's work *Après Canguilhem* (2010), from the point of view that the extreme quantification of health after Big Data has a double sense of being objective and equally contributing to the creation of normative claims and evaluation, like the "average" patient or the "statistically deviant", etc. From the middle of the 20th century, the biomedical sciences proceeded to important developments; in parallel, there have been major concerns that modern medicine was attached to a naturalist account of the normal and the pathological. The critique revolved around issues that, beyond their medical dimension, also concern sociology, history, anthropology. Examples include Thomas Szazs and his study on alcoholism, Richard Green on homosexuality, Allan Barnes on menopause, Tristam Engelhardt on masturbation, and, finally, Tristam Engelhadt and Arthur Caplan on aging.[256] The conception of the disease as biological normativity was proposed by Georges Canguilhem, against the conception of the patho-

---

[256]   Élodie Giroux, *Après Canguilhem* (Paris: Presses universitaires de France, 2010), 7.

logical as deficiency or surplus of biological factor, promoted by François Broussais. Therefore, we could not speak for "statistical deviance", the holistic approach of Lennart Nordenfelt, which underlines the ability of the patient to act, considered by Élodie Giroux as a moderate normativism, and finally theanalytic and bio-statistical method of Christopher Boorse, which, as we will see, asserts that the theory of "statistical deviance" is neither necessary nor sufficient to define disease. Normativity holds in its core the idea that disease is a social construct while naturalism proclaims that a scientific and objective concept of disease exists.

Giroux proposes that in order to understand the notion of Canguilhem's biological normativity, we should first take note of the fact that he speaks about a biological individuality, in the sense that the organism is the entity that corresponds better to the notion of individual, rather than the cell or the society. Canguilhem proceeds to a broad clarification of notions, like the distinction between health and normality, and pathology in distinction with abnormality. The pathological is not the absence of the norm, but a restrictive normativity, a norm of a life which is inferior. The disease is defined as "a state with a negative value for a living individual". Health, on the other hand, is the vital opposite of the pathological, described as the capability of living beings to recover from disease, stress, and the modifications of the environment they live in by creating their proper norms of living. Subsequently, health is a superior norm of the living.[257] The objectivity of the pathological lies in two pillars for Canguilhem: biological normality and individuality. What distinguishes the physiological from the pathological is not an objective reality of a physico-chemical type, but rather a biological value. The living prefers life to death and health to disease; it chooses and selects. The living favors certain norms or values of life; consequently, it maintains itself and is individualized. For this reason, regarding individuality, for Canguilhem, it is not proper to speak about diseased organs and tissues, or cells, but rather about a single diseased individual. Contrary to Claude Bernard, Canguilhem conceives medicine not as the science of normal functions, but as a science of stabilized modes of life.[258]

Nordenfelt follows a different pathway to Canguilhem.[259] For him, illness is not connected with a restrictive normativity, but is rather an

---

[257]   Élodie Giroux, *Après Canguilhem*, 28.
[258]   Ibid., 23–24.
[259]   Ibid., 58.

ability. He continues the work of Caroline Whitbeck and Ingmar Pörn, who has been influenced by the ideas of Talcott Parsons, who gives a notion of health as the ability of the individual to perform the social roles and tasks through which it has been socialized. Illness affects the ability of action, while health and welfare are seen as the ability of the individual in the second order[260] to fulfill its vital scopes (the minimal scopes which are necessary for achieving a minimal welfare). This ability is a type of possibility for action, determined by the internal factors of body and mind of the agent.

Nordenfelt's holistic approach has some discrete points of reference. First, it is an approach in which concepts of health and disease are more centered upon the individual; therefore, the criteria for health coexist with sociological and psychological perspectives. This is exemplified in his view that a healthy person should be good and function in a social context. Second, the notion of health has a logical priority over the disease. He asserts that it is logically impossible to define disease without making reference to health; this is linked with contemporary medical practice which aims for public health and preventive medicine and promotes health in general. Third, he favors a positive conception of health that is not only the absence of disease, but is connected with well-being, happiness, and action, or better, ability. [261]

The theory of bio-statistics and analytics (applied to the levels of the whole organism), conceived by Christopher Boorse, is an attempt to provide an objective definition of health, far from relativism and normativity, and has at least two discrete stages of development.[262] The first (1975) was to clarify the terms **disease**, **illness** and **sickness**. **Disease** is the objective (medical) state, **illness** refers to **being ill**, and finally **sickness** is the social dimension of **being an ill**. Health for him has a **negative** dimension, which is the absence of disease, without completely excluding the possibility of a **positive** character, if we consider the en-

---

[260]   Nordenfelt takes the example of a political refugee who was capable of cultivating the land in his country of origin so as to take care of his family, but incapable of doing that work in his host country. This in any case means that he became ill in his new environment. A person may be incapable in a first order of fulfilling a certain action, but in a second order potentially capable of fulfilling it. See: Elodie Giroux, "Philosophie de la medicine" in *Précis de philosophie des sciences*, ed. Anouk Barberousse, Denis Bonnay, and Mikaël Cozic (Paris: Vuibert, 2015), 420.

[261]   Élodie Giroux, *Après Canguilhem*, 56–57.

[262]   Élodie Giroux, ""Philosophie de la Medicine" in *Précis De Philosophie Des Sciences*, ed. Anouk Barberousse, Denis Bonnay, and Mikaël Cozic (Paris: Vuibert, 2015), 417–21.

hancement of health while we recover from a disease. Boorse, in order to avoid any possible relativism occurring from the above is led to an objective, non-normative, value-free definition of health. He asserts that on the theoretical level of physiology, the approach to the normal and the pathological does not necessitate the involvement of social and subjective values or norms. Western medicine, first and foremost, proclaims that the normal is the natural and health is conformity to the design of the species; consequently, health and disease are notions which are opposed and exclusive.[263] In the opposite direction, pathology uses a theoretical concept of disease, which is independent of the clinical practice and the values which it introduces.

The second stage (1977) provides a broader definition of disease, far from the theory of statistical deviance, which has seven characteristics:[264]

Value: Health in general is desirable and it is connected with physical well-being. On the other hand, there are conditions which can restrict well-being that are not diseases, e.g., below average height or strength, which we could not distinguish from diseases on grounds of negative value alone.

Treatment by physicians: Treatment can be considered neither necessary nor sufficient for something to be a disease. There may be a broad list of cases that surely demand treatment, or cases that cannot be treated—e.g., certain forms of cancer. On the other hand, procedures like circumcision or cosmetic surgery are not characterized as interventions aiming to cure a disease by any medical text.

Statistical Normality: Health in medical textbooks is conceived of as normal, while diseases or pathological conditions are abnormal. A form of describing normality is statistical normality with a certain range of normal variation. In Boorse's functional account, statistical normality fails to categorize a condition either as normal or as pathological if we consider the example of red hair or the O blood type.

Pain, suffering, and discomfort: According to Boorse this conception prioritizes medical praxis rather than medical theory, an idea briefly stated above. In cases, for example, of asymptomatic diseases, there is no pain or discomfort. In contrast, pain can also occur during normal processes like childbirth.

---

[263] Ibid., 411.
[264] Christopher Boorse, "Health as a Theoretical Concept," *Philosophy of Science* 44, no. 4 (1977):542–73.

Disability: Disability is often linked with the loss of the capacity to perform a task, even a vital task, and in most cases is considered painful. However, according to Boorse, it could be so broad that it could include minor skin diseases, e.g., athlete's foot, or disabilities like myopia. Furthermore, it is normal for an adult to walk, something that is not normal for babies.

Adaptation: From the perspective of a biologist, standard abilities of organisms are adaptations to their environment; this is not synonymous with Darwinian fitness or reproductive success. Boorse refers to Ryle as the prominent supporter of this view of adaptation and concludes that Ryle's normality is more like practical normality which does not demand medical attention; it is not a theoretical normality which implies freedom from disease. Abilities may improve well-being in a particular environment, but their lack is not always pathological. Consequently, it is not "pathological for a person X in environment E", but "bad for X in E".

Homeostasis: Boorse claims that the importance of homeostasis, as defended mainly by Claude Bernard and Walter Cannon, cannot be that of a general model of proper biological function and equilibrium. Some processes may be homeostatic, but if we consider, for example, perception, locomotion, and reproduction, they are linked with an upset of equilibrium. Consequently, diseases like deafness, limb paralysis, or sterility could not be homeostatic problems.

According to Boorse, the model that he proposes has some success and some anomalies. As for the successes: 1) it explains the divergence between judgments of defense and those of desirability and treatability; 2) it captures the medical view of traits with a continuous distribution in the population; 3) it makes health judgments independent of the gross output of the organism; and 4) biologists can apply the notion of disease as readily to animals and plants. As for the anomalies, they are related to two kinds of diseases: 1) structural diseases, excluding entries in the nomenclature that are purely structural disorders; e.g., dextrocardia and calcification of pineal gland; and 2) universal diseases such as dental cavities and leg irritation.[265]

In any case, statistical normality still plays a vital role in Boorse's theory, but it is seen in the spectrum of biological function. Pathologies are internal states which reduce a functional capacity below the typical levels of the human species, health is the statistical normality of a mal-

---

[265]   Christopher Boorse, "Health as a Theoretical Concept".

function, and finally, practical health is the absence of a disease that can be treated.

Medical nihilism, in general, is the view that we should have little reliance on the effectiveness of medical interventions. Jacob Stegenga not only thinks this of conditions with no special treatment—e.g., certain forms of cancer or Parkinson's disease—but focuses more on the efficacy of methods like metadata analysis and randomized control trials that are considered the gold standard for contemporary medicine. In any case, this stance, which is based both on empirical research and epistemological aspects, should not be confused with anti-scientific or dangerous views like anti-vaccine campaigns and implausible alternatives such as homeopathy, etc.[266] In our analysis we will focus only on the second chapter of his book *Medical Nihilism* titled "Effectiveness of medical interventions", because it is related to the debate between naturalism and normativism. He proposes a hybridist account of health and disease which argues that there is a constitutive causal basis of disease, as well as a normative basis.

Stegenga starts from Boorse's naturalist approach, which proposes a mechanistic scheme, in which disease is a failure of parts of the body to perform biological functions that are statistically normal, and whose ultimate aim is contribution to survival and reproduction. Consequently, health is the ability of one's physiological system to function at typical efficiency, while disease is the opposite. The inability to function at typical efficiency is, for Stegenga, the causal basis of a disease. The target of a medical intervention that reestablishes this physiological function is called a causal target of effectiveness. A classical example is the exogenous administration of insulin in diabetes.[267]

Contrary to a naturalist account of health and disease, Stegenga gives the example of homosexuality, which is no longer considered a disease and, of course, is not related to a reduction of biological function below typical efficiency. Another major problem is the determination of class of reference, through which normality is accessed because someone's biological function may be within a normal range, but in other cases outside this classification. This fact may be appealing to non-biological considerations of normality, thus proposing a value-laden and not a value-free conception of a disease. Stegenga gives the example of depression to clarify this fact.

[266]   Jacob Stegenga, *Medical Nihilism* (Oxford: Oxford University Press, 2018), 17.
[267]   Jacob Stegenga, *Medical Nihilism*, 26.

Stegenga unfolds his thoughts on normativism, following the analysis of Rachel Cooper, who conceives of disease as a bad thing; thus, the affected person may be unlucky and probably medically treated. Cooper refers to the statistical rareness of red hair color by arguing that it may be outside a typical color reference if we consider the naturalist claim, but is not something harmful. In other words, red hair is not a bad thing. Stegenga assigns the requirement of a state to be disvalued in order for it to be a normative basis of disease. [268]

The normative target of effectiveness is achieved when a medical intervention is considered effective if it improves a harmful effect of a disease. Some states that are considered harmful do not have a constitutive causal basis—e.g., wealth inequality and poverty. So, there should be a mechanism to distinguish disease from states evaluated as bad or harmful. Normativists support the view that a harmful state can be considered a disease if it is disvalued by physicians and not by, for example, welfare counselors. A second prescription is that a state should be medically treatable. For example, diabetes is treatable while poverty is not.

Stegenga proposes a hybrid account for the resolution of the problems between naturalism and normativism.[269] Disease, according to hybridism, must hold two positions. First, a state must be biologically dysfunctional and second, this dysfunction must be harmful. It is a view which preserves both the causal basis of the disease and the normative basis. The hybridist view can be seen more easily in the context of psychiatry. Stegenga refers to the current DSMV, which states that although brain-based dysfunctions are not completely understood, they are an essential part of defining behavioral, cognitive, and emotional symptom syndromes; thus, there is a causal basis of disease from a naturalist perspective. He also refers to social anxiety, which can be treated with the drug paroxetine. With a naturalist approach, if panoxetil can treat social anxiety, it can satisfy a causal basis. But from another point of view, social anxiety may be caused by social norms and values that can harm the individual; thus, there are also aspects of a value-laden or normative basis for a disease. In any case, hybridism aims at cure and care. If medical intervention satisfies the causal target of effectiveness, then the interaction can be used to cure; if it satisfies the normative target of effectiveness, it can be used to care.

---

[268]   Jacob Stegenga, *Medical Nihilism*,30.
[269]   Jacob Stegenga, *Medical Nihilism*, 34.

Conclusions

In this chapter, we focused our attention to the omic revolution. Our purpose was to present its respected contribution to precision medicine, therapeutics, and diagnostics. This was further illuminated and broadened by an overview of the existing bibliography concerning mainly preventive models of several diseases (coronary disease, mammary and ovarian cancer, and stomach ulcers and cancer). Big Data was first characterized by the so called three Vs (volume, velocity, and variety). We then described the transition to five Vs because the two new characteristics value, and veracity or validity, encapsulate its economic and ethical dimensions. We posed the question of how knowledge acquisition can be done through Big Data, something that can also have an epistemological dimension. Consequently, we decided to present the nine-step Knowledge Discovery in Database (KDD) model of data mining knowledge acquisition. Beyond the nine-step KDD data mining, knowledge obtained from Big Data demands statistical analysis in order to be quantified. Therefore, we continued with the presentation of the methods used in algorithmic statistical analysis of Big Data (supervised, non-supervised, and semi-supervised methods). Beyond the statistical analysis and quantification, there are methods of knowledge acquisition, through the correlation of data, so we proceeded to the definitions of machine and deep learning in order to clarify how they work and how they are modeled. But, beyond their modeling, we saw how they can apply in medicine, for what purposes they are used, if there are efficacy issues and limitations, and for this reason we enumerated several cases based on particular research. Since biomechanics (the omic revolution) and bioinformatics (all the tools of Big Data generation and management just mentioned above) lead to a more precise knowledge of the disease on a molecular basis, we presented the need of a new categorization of disease and the model that could be implemented. The taxonomy of a disease is an epistemological issue, in which doctors and biologists focus their attention throughout the years proposing different approaches and criteria for categorization; we selected crucial historical facts in order to reveal the difficulties and the change of perspective which gradually led us to contemporary models. Big Data, beyond its practicality, also has certain limits, concerning both its nature (the curse of dimensionality, missing values) and its application (data in relation to in-vivo parameters). Another important epistemological issue we posed was what happens with the so-called randomized control trial, which is considered the gold standard for contemporary medicine; we decided to expose its limits. These limits were approached as a general rethinking and not from the point of view of a total critique and skepticism. Data-driven and hypothesis-driven scientific models have been seen in light of important epistemological issues arising, like the new emerging empiricism of Big Data, admitting that correlation is enough. This empiricism may be considered as a paradigmatic change from the supporters of the information revolution, but as we showed, it has certain deficiencies. One major deficiency is epistemic opacity; recognizing this problem, we focused on models proposed for its resolution. Reconsidering all the above issues and their impact on medicine, we claimed that a new approach is needed, combining the relevance of logic in medical praxis which assures the patient's safety (abductive reasoning over the deductive and inductive) with a generic conception of epistemology able to deal with the interdisciplinarity of the various scientific fields through which Big Data is generated. Finally, a rethinking of Levinas and Derrida is related to our basic theoretical assumptions when we turn to medical praxis. In our last section we emphasized the debate between naturalism and normativism, which helped us to overview the various definitions of health and disease in a context of Big Data (the average patient and statistical abnormality and deviance).

Chapter 6:
Information Society and a New Form of Embodiment

Introduction

At the dawn of the 21st century, the body and, subsequently, embodiment, had attracted the interest of the academic community. The body is not approached merely as a physical entity but in relation with the social, cultural, political, and economic terrain. The positivist assumption of classical sociology, which claims that the body belongs primarily to biology, has collapsed. We could enumerate several instances in which the interweaving of the body with fields that surpass its biological limits can give us a clearer view of the so-called "turn to the body" or "new materialism". Technological progress in biology, medicine, genomics, cognitive science, and neuroscience provided valuable knowledge about the way our bodies function or interact with others and the environment. Furthermore, the rise of civil movements around sexual liberation and the recognition of sexual and racial minorities placed the body as the keystone of contemporary struggles and debates over embodied oppression of different kinds—e.g., patriarchy, rape, domestic violence, racially excluded bodies, etc. Current trends and programs of personal enhancement or human transformation, like specialized diets or cosmetic surgery, concern embodiment as a consumer lifestyle. Finally, contemporary transnational capitalism more and more seeks flexible working bodies with the appropriate biometric and social characteristics so that maximum functionality will be achieved. With respect to the crucial issues above, a new interdisciplinary academic field has been established, that of "body studies". Today, there are plenty of undergraduate and postgraduate programs, as well as journals, devoted to the field.

In this chapter we will focus upon new media technologies, informatization, and digitality, and how they affect embodiment. Hubert Dreyfus proclaims the risk-free aspect of digitality. Physical presence can be accompanied by a certain vulnerability of the self, which in a digital world is reduced or eliminated because there is no commitment and action.[270] Sherry Turkle speaks about a break of physical interconnected-

---

[270]   Cf. Hubert Dreyfus, *On the Internet* (New York: Routledge, 2008).

ness and the loneliness of our body-experiential world in the digital environment.[271] Anna Munster suggests that in digital embodiment we do not have an immediate connection with the body as itself but the relation lies more between the body and the digital interface.[272]

We will refer to at least six categories of bodies or embodiment in the information society. The first category is that of *bodily governance.* Issues like data collection from the internet will be exposed, which are connected not only with the websites that users visit but with the clicks or the average time spent on websites and complete tracking records. In comparison with the increasing violation of privacy, alternative plug-ins and applications that have been created and raise questions about the explicated digital world like *AdNauseam,* or redefine the relationship between the digital and the physical, like *I'm Getting Arrested,* will contribute to our understanding of technologies and counter-technologies which fight over personal data collection. Furthermore, after 9/11, or more recently after the emergence of ISIS and the Islamic State, bodily governance has expanded to the extreme control of public spaces with monitoring systems and specialized systems of surveillance (fingerprint collection, voice recognition, DNA sample collection, etc.)

The second category is that of the *transforming body.* The *transforming body* may refer to organ transplantation, which reveals the vital issue of the biological limits of our bodies, prosthetics, which reshape in many cases our experiential perception of space and the environment, and plastic surgery. Plastic surgery is mainly linked with the pursuit of the dominant perception of beauty and aesthetic values which are formed nowadays mostly through advertising and social media and go together with the consumerist lifestyle. Plastic surgery has also been used in order for racial oppression to be eliminated. Immigrants coming from eastern countries perform surgeries of the eyelid so that their facial characteristics are compatible with the western; in this case, we have a fusion of *bodily governance* and a *transforming body.*

The third category is that of *virtual bodies.* Virtual bodies concern either our placement in virtual environments with the use of special gloves, glasses, or catsuits and our interaction with them, or platforms where our embodied virtual experience is achieved through avatars. In

---

[271]   Cf. Sherry Trakle, *Alone Together* (New York: Basic Books, a member of the Perseus Books Group, 2012). Jacques Quintin, "Organ Transplantation and Meaning of Life: The Quest for Self Fulfilment," *Med Health Care and Philos*, no. 16 (2012).
[272]   Cf. Anna Munster, *Materializing New Media* (Hanover, N.H.: Dartmouth College Press, 2012).

the first case, dilemmas around our split of physical and virtual body occur, giving the essence of a disembodied experience. In the latter case, the debate revolves around socialization and how it is formed in these platforms, or how we choose to project our virtual avatar in relation with our true selves and, consequently, how our identity is perceived. Identity and its perception are also connected with a more applied or practical issue, that of the various options which the platforms offer to visualize our avatars—e.g., masculine, feminine, or animal form, and first person, third person, mirrored self-angle, etc.

The fourth category is that of *medical bodies*. Modern medical approaches seem to question the dominant biomedical model, which is based on strict evidence-based data and objective criteria. There is much concern about the subjective feeling of the patient, how his life changes in relation to his problem, and the impact on his relatives and workplace. We can grasp a more human-based view which accounts for social and psychological factors involved in the therapeutic process. Furthermore, physicians do not only prescribe drugs and implement protocols, but they also give information and advice about a healthy lifestyle and appropriate consumption habits and propose patterns of organizing the social and the working space. Progress has also been made in the way modern medicine treats people with special needs as well as elders. They are not the "disabled" or "aged" bodies anymore, but active agents who participate in social activities and are worthy of welfare and ethical practices. New technologies for mobility and mental problems play a vital role as well as establish the field of gerontology. To sum up, the body is conceived of as a holistic project rather than simply a diseased body needing to be cured.

The last category is that of *sexual bodies*. In this section we will discuss new theories in feminism and gender studies which deal with the performativity of gender, as well as the new forms of sexual experience between human and non-human entities like machines and robots, and intercourse in cyber-environments either with physical presence or through avatars.

In the sixth category, *transhuman bodies*, we strive towards a general outline of what is called transhumanism, the origins as well the theories which gave birth to the current perception of the term. We focus on the anthropological aspects of transhumanism, mainly those of Andy Clack, who reconsiders prosthetics when it comes to the body and also to our cognitive systems, from an evolutionary point of view in which humans now incorporate the tools that they learned to use throughout evolution. Then we look upon the important issue of how new technologies, mainly those centered in biomedicine and biotechnology, may not only be used for general well-being or a good life, but as chances for a triumph against death, resituating the human as an almost immortal being. We pose short problems, like the immorality of a possible immortality. We also deal with the theory of Rossi Braidotti, who asks if our general human-centered world-view supersedes other living entities. Are there auto-poietic processes to general evolution? Is the human subject something static or is it decentered and nomadic? Finally, we expose the various theories regarding superintelligence and singularity (Vernor Vinge, Ray Kurzweil, Nick Bostrom) to ask what that powerful technology, which surpasses human intelligence and is also capable of imitating emotions and feelings, is and what its risks are. What does it mean for evolution?

6.1 Bodily Governance

Following Shilling,[273] classical sociology and political philosophy provide us with remarkable theory on *bodily governance*. Max Weber, with his diligent analysis of Protestant ethics, presents how religious beliefs shape the bodily identities and behavior of individuals. He links the long working hours as the dogma of rational capitalism with the immersion of the workers in a sinful pleasure and a pursuit of worldly signs of election and entering heavenly life. Nobert Elias describes how etiquette books from the Renaissance onwards provided detailed codes of body management and prohibitions which regulated courtesy and were used as the measure of differentiation of the relative worth of people. Jeremy Bentham proposed the *panopticon* model of an institutional building and a system of control. In this model, the prisoners are placed in the center, without the ability to tell whether they are being inspected or not, and a guard observes them from the periphery. Michel Foucault, in his theory of discipline and punishment, refers to the *panopticon* model as a method that promoted prisoners' self-control so that they could become productive members of society. Foucault analyzed the changes that took place in the European penal system during modernity and thus gave us a compelling view of how structures function through forms of bio-power which imprint themselves on and within bodies. Foucault defines these

---

[273]   Chris Shilling, "The Rise of Body Studies and Embodiment," *Horizons in Humanities and Social Sciences*, no.1 (2016): 22–46.

practices of the modern state as "an explosion of numerous and diverse techniques for achieving the subjugations of bodies and the control of populations."[274]

Data collections, through tracking records of searching machines, social media, credit cards, and insurance companies today form a *post-panopticon* model. The new model is dispersed and diffused almost everywhere, leaving aside the strict locality of the *panopticon*. Furthermore, new social media allow the many (the many users) to inspect the few (the economic elites, or VIPs); in Zygmunt Bauman's conception this can be called as a *synopticon* model.[275] But if we consider the fact that data in most cases is under the authority of big economic institutions, we could admit that the model turns into a *revesred synopticon*.[276] Bauman's assumptions regarding the liquefaction of modernity—by which the world of solid, heavy structures is changing into an infinite set of flows—together with his *synopticon*, lead David Lyon to speak of *liquid surveillance*. According to Lyon,

> Surveillance not only creeps and seeps, it also flows. It is on the move, globally and locally. The means of tracing and tracking the mobilities of the twenty-first century are "going global" in the sense that connections are increasingly sought between one system and another. The quest for harmonization of, for example, machine-readable travel documents so that systems are "interoperable" between as well as within countries actually harmonizes the technologic of IT with the political economy of globalization.[277]

As a response to extreme electronic surveillance, projects like the *AdNauseam* plugin have been elaborated. *AdNauseam* functions similarly to an ad-blocker, but with some remarkable differences. It obfuscates user data by clicking all the links on the visited page provided by the ad platform and then creates a large set of data that is useless to the tracking services. The project aims not to go against advertising itself but to challenge us to become aware of electronic surveillance and privacy in the digital realm. Another interesting case is that of the application *I'm Getting Arrested*. It emerged through the Occupy Wall Street movement and

---

[274]   Michel Foucault, *The History of Sexuality, vol. 1* (London: Penguin Books, 1998), 140.

[275]   Cf. Zygmunt Bauman and David Lyon, *Liquid Surveillance: A Conversation* (Cambridge: Polity Press, 2016).

[276]   For more about the reversed synopticon model, please see Alexander Gungov, "Real Semblance Flourishing in Post-Consumerist Society," *Sofia Philosophical Review*, vol. VII, no. 2, 2013.

[277]   David Lyon, "Liquid Surveillance: The Contribution of Zygmunt Bauman to Surveillance Studies," *International Political Sociology*, no. 4 (2010): 323–38.

has also been used in other civil mobilizations. It works simply when someone is arrested; it sends a pre-formatted text to multiple receivers— e.g., friends, lawyers, and journalists. Through this project, we can understand how a technological advantage can promote objectives in the physical world and challenge existing power structures.[278]

The last cases of bodily governance that we would like to present are *biological and neurological citizenship* and the *collection of biometric data.* Chris Shilling,[279] citing the writers below, asserts that the first notion implies that in order for someone to be a citizen who is ethically acceptable they should dispose "received facts" which come from science and medicine. Hereditary problems and risks associated with following a certain lifestyle, such as alcohol consumption, are all accounted for in building the profile of the citizen who can stand as the ethical paradigm in society. According to the anthropologist Kaushik S. Rajan, individuals become "patients in waiting".[280] The patient in waiting promotes the economic value of physical and mental health as expressed in the individual, in health care services, and in national productivity. Because of a terrorist menace and possible social turbulence, after 9/11 and ISIS, as well as after the refugee crisis that broke out, we had the creation of alien bodies which had to be meticulously registered and monitored. Fingerprint, voice, and iris recognition, DNA sample collection at airports and refugee camps, CCTV monitoring systems in public spaces, and undercover police operations can reveal how our bodies become passwords.[281] From another perspective, Giorgio Agamben describes the collection of biometric data as being similar to the tattooing of Jews during the Holocaust. Biometrics turn the human persona into a bare body. Agamben distinguishes the use of the two ancient Greek terms which indicate "life", *zoe,* which is the life common to animals and humans, and *bios*, which describes human life with its meanings and purposes. The contemporary state shapes a new bio-political relationship between citizens and reduces their life to purely the biological, given above with the term *zoe*, with a parallel reduction of their human characteristics (*bios*). Biometrics contribute to this remarkable shift.[282]

---

[278]   T. Dufva, and M. Dufva, "*Grasping the future of the digital society*," Futures, no. 107 (2019):17–28.

[279]   Chris Shilling, "The Rise of Body Studies and Embodiment," *Horizons In Humanities And Social Sciences*, no. 1 (2016): 22–46.

[280]   Cf. Kaushik Sunder Rajan, *Biocapital* (Durham: Duke University Press, 2007).

[281]   Ann Davis, "The Body as Password". *Wired*, January 7, 1997, https://www.wired.com /1997/07/biometrics-, last accessed, January 25, 2020.

[282]   Cf. Gorgio Agamben, *Homo Sacer* (Stanford, Calif.: Stanford University Press, 1998).

6.2 Transforming Bodies

Our bodies, in their physical aspect, are under continuous transformation. The chemical composition of our tissues changes over time; our cells regenerate. If we also consider the social impact of our bodily changes, the growth of our muscles depends on our dietary habits, our kind of work, etc. Lynda Birke calls on us to rethink our biological bodies under the spectrum of transformation or, better, the possibility of transformation, in distinction with the stability of the genes that certain theories propose. We do not "unfold" by expressing a predetermined genetic sequence as it is coded in the DNA, from the moment the semen fuses with the ovum; this is in no case a micro-version of our future selves. There are other ways for someone to approach a human *being in a process of becoming*, like the growth of the embryo which actively takes place.[283] The embryo actively reshapes its environment, though it can be seen as a self-organized entity rather than a passive victim of its genetic inheritance.[284]

Organ transplantations and donations raise a critical question regarding the alteration of our subjective experience concerning our bodily image, our conceptualization of life, and our natural limits. The very fundamental essence of medicine is also under reconsideration: does medicine exist to care for us and to heal and relieve us from pain, or does it deal with the improvement of the human race? The ethical dilemmas that occur emphasize consent, the definition of death, and the rules that regulate organ distribution, and ask whether it has merely become a business affair.[285] In another part of his analysis, Shilling[286] claims that David Harvey suggests that we live a period of primitive accumulation. This can be envisaged both from the human slavery that still exists and also by the growth of "transplant trafficking", the "global billion-dollar criminal industry which transports fresh organs from living and dead to the affluent and medically insured mobile transplant patients".[287]

---

[283] Lynd Birke, "Soma Kai Viologia," In *Viokoinonikoties Ta Oria Tou Somatos Diepistimonikes Prosegisis* (Athens: Nisos, 2014), 149–59.

[284] Cf. Brian Carey Goodwin, *How the Leopard Changed its Spots* (Princeton, N.J: Princeton University Press, 2001).

[285] Jacques, Quintin, "Organ Transplantation and Meaning Of Life: The Quest For Self Fulfilment," Med Health Care And Philos, no. 16 (2012): 565–74.

[286] Chris Shilling, "The Rise of Body Studies and Embodiment".

[287] David Harvey, "The new imperialism. Accumulation by dispossession," *Social Register*, no. 40 (2004): 63–67

In the information society, new forms of organ transplantation have emerged, such as 3D-printed biomaterials. They are biomaterials technically reproduced layer by layer to create tissue-like structures that imitate real tissues, with the use of fresh cells (in most cases stem cells) collected from the patient and growth factors, known as bioink. The biomaterials can consist of parts of body tissues up to fully printed organs.[288] 3D-printed biomaterials and organs promise to solve some of the major problems that conventional organ transplantations have, such as histocompatibility and the following immunosuppressive medication, which is prescribed to the patients in order for the transplant not to be rejected, and is accompanied by various side effects, the long queues most patients face as candidates for a transplant, and, finally, problems which concern donation, distribution, or even organ trafficking. Beyond the promises 3D-printed biomaterials bring, there are also ethical issues related to experimental testing on humans, the risks of significant harm associated with testing, as well as the possible irreversibility, the loss of treatment opportunity, the lack of a specific framework for regulation and testing, and—finally—the high cost of the biomaterials produced, combined with the fact that they are offered only to those who can afford them.[289]

Prostheses or prosthetics used in amputees or in some cases paralytics is another form of body transformation, as Murray,[290] citing the authors below, argues that these people lose their conceptual links to the world which are connected to their very existence.[291] They also face problems concerning the "authorship" of their actions, since they may lose the ability to control their movements or their body in general and this can affect their "ownership or identification of the self with the body".[292] Phantom phenomena can also appear in patients who make use of prosthetics. Their experiences concerning their missing parts of the body can be regarded as either painful and giving the essence of someone locked in the same position, or more rewarding, providing the capability of movement sometimes under the patient's conscious control. Merleau-Ponty contributed to our understanding of phantom phenomena. He con-

---

[288]   Chana Sirota, "3D Organ Printing," The Science Journal of The Lander College of Arts and Sciences, no. 10 (2006).

[289]   Gilbert, Frederic, Cathal D. O'Connell, Tajanka Mladenovska, and Susan Dodds, "Print Me an Organ? Ethical And Regulatory Issues Emerging From 3D Bioprinting in Medicine," Science and Engineering Ethics, no.24 (2017).

[290]   D, Murray C, "Towards a Phenomenology of the Body in Virtual Reality," Research in Philosophy and Technology, (2000): 149–73.

[291]   Cf. Murphy Robert, The Body Silent (London:J.M. Dent and Sons Ltd, 1997).

[292]   Cf. Rom Hare, Physical Being (Oxford: Blackwell, 1991).

siders that these phenomena are a result of the "being-in-the world"; patients in a way remain open to a customary world and retain the practicality enjoyed before mutilation. We could speak for a separation between two bodies, the customary and the body "at this moment".[293] Plastic surgery, beyond the obvious changes in our appearance, brings changes in tactility and proprioception. In breast augmentation, for example, rude touch and light pressure sensation are affected, while in eyelid surgeries, we have a greater scope for our vision (sight); thus, in general, we can speak about subjective changes which are deeply connected to embodiment and do not solely concern the transformation of the body under the spectrum of aestheticization of everyday life and the pursuit of a dominant lifestyle.

6.3 Virtual Bodies

Referring again to Murray, virtual technologies and the way we immerse ourselves in virtual environments have progressed in time. At the start we had the use of virtual glasses in which vision was the main link between our physical and virtual body, and then specially designed gloves that covered parts of the body, mainly torsos, gave the opportunity of a more embodied experience, since beyond vision the sensations of grasping or touching have been incorporated in our virtual experience. Today we have even more advanced methods, like catsuits which cover the whole body and provide full motion detection and enable the animation of the virtual body viewable via a head-mounted visual display. We can speak consequently of the participation of almost all the main parts of the body which provide sensation. Frank Biocca speaks for a virtual experience becoming all-embodying, and even re-embodying, but he also raises the critical question of how VR peripherals block the sensory impressions from physical reality.[294] Apart from the blocking of our physical experience, neo-Cartesian readings of virtual (dis)embodiment and mind-body duality have been proposed, since VR has predominantly visual characteristics and can be considered as an optical technology. Users immersed in virtual environments may characterize their experience as leaving their bodies behind, or "disappearing", giving "way to the dis-

---

[293]   Cf. Merleau-Ponty, Maurice, *Phenomenology of Perception: An Introduction* (London: Routledge, 2011).

[294]   Cf. Frank, Biocca, and Levy Mark *Communication Applications of Virtual Reality* (Hillsdale: Lawrence Erlbaum Associates, 2015).

embodied traveler, the astral projectionist, the 'interface data cow-boy'".[295]

The other form of virtual embodiment which we would like to discuss is that of avatars, which are a visual-virtual representation of our bodies in digital platforms which permit both the interaction with the digital environment and the users. Our primary concern regarding these forms of embodiment is how the users choose to socialize and what the options of communication, signs, and language are that a platform can provide, imitating customary and everyday forms of intersubjective interaction. In *Dreamscape,* for example, one of the best-known digital platforms, the users can indicate their presence with a greeting which is performed with a wave or jump. The communication or "speaking" between the users is achieved through real-time dialogue via text bubbles that appear overhead; the expressiveness of the avatar is also used to display emotions, usually through facial expressions or movements. Phenomena of crossing boundaries and invasion of personal space can also appear. In these cases, placement of the avatars face-to-face, with the attributing facial expressions and dialogue, can signify anger or dispute; on the contrary, when avatars touch each other, it may express intimacy or friendship. There are also more formal codes with which the avatars can signify, like common dress codes or names between couples or partners, groups, etc. Users also participate in social occasions, like a public funeral of a possibly dead user (a user abandoning the platform); this is usually performed by the users gathering in a circle around the avatar of the perished user and with facial expressions of sorrow; they may even drop flowers, etc. There were also cases in which online religious services were provided in the Dreamscape platform. A fair-sized Christian community held worship events in which people would raise their avatar arms, dance, and assume many other forms quite similar to some offline behaviors.[296]

Existing isochronally in both the real and the virtual worlds, something called a "bifurcated self" challenges us to rethink whether the two bodies (real and virtual) inhabit both spaces equally if our consciousness (even more, the part of the consciousness coming from the embodying experiencing) also participates equally. Do we remain ourselves during

---

[295]   Cf. Bogard William, *The Simulation of Surveillance: Hypercontrol in Telematic Societies* (New York: Cambridge University Press, 2016).

[296]   Jacquelyn Ford Morie, "Performing in (Virtual) Spaces: Embodiment and Being in Virtual Environments," *International Journal of Performance Arts and Digital Media,* no. 3 (2006): 123–38.

VR immersion, or do we have a more performing role, as in theater or films? Are the two states of embodiment diacritical or complementary? There are various types of visualization in virtual environments. A first-person angle or no avatar is no representation at all; the environment appears as seen through our eyes. This type mainly permits the user to stay in touch with his inner conception of the self. The mirrored self-type provides a view similar to video camera capturing. The mirrored self is a dualistic form; we have a separation between the physical and virtual body spatially but not temporally. Graphical personification is different from the mirrored self; in this case, we have a graphical representation of the body which appears to occupy the same space as our physical presence would. This representation corresponds to our own body since the 3D creator can select whether this is a representation of a humanoid, an animal far from our typical human representation, or of a single gender, for instance. Are we projecting only male human bodies regardless of our real gender? Third-person is more common in video games than VR; in this type our embodying experience is placed outside our perceptual self. We are more like observers in a phenomenal dichotomy, in which we cannot define if we ourselves or others control us.[297]

6.4 Medical Bodies

Modern medicine seems to make a variable turn; the former purely material, diseased body, which needed to be cured, is now a body in which the subjective narratives of the patient and social infiltration may reflect better its essence. In the last 30 years, there has been a call for a more human-based approach, considering the patient not as someone deviating from evidence-based golden standards, but as a personality which actively interacts during his healing process. A patient does not only follow the prescriptions of the physician and improve the parameters that define the severity of his condition, but also cultivates a subjective narrative of his experience and tries to establish new methods of interaction with his natural and social environment. New medical models that question the biomedical model have been proposed by various theorists, such as the biopsychosocial, the infomedical and the model of personal narrative. The first model, introduced by George L. Engel, focuses on the deficiencies of the biomedical model and proposes methods of correction, like the consideration of an active disease or manifestation of an illness as a

---

[297]   Ibid.

phenomenon with complex interactions of factors, not as only starting from a primary cause (recognition of multiple causation). He considers the psychological, social, and cultural factors which may be involved in the experiencing of the symptoms of a disease in general (recognition of various levels of activity) and, finally, how a disease varies individually.[298] The infomedical model suggested by Laurence Foss explores how sociocultural carriers of information called memes can interact with a disease, and especially with anorexia nervosa. In this case, an image of or belief about the ideal weight of the body functions as a "mimetic vector" and "programs" the metabolism in a complementary way with the genetic programming[299]. The narrative model seeks to describe the process of getting ill or recovering and may uncover alternative or new therapeutic options by accounting for the personal experience of a patient. It addresses existential and social qualities like emotions (pain, sorrow, despair, and hope), which often accompany illness, or emphasizes how the life of patient or his relatives can change, for instance, with the abandonment of a lifestyle or activities which he enjoyed in the past, and the care that should be provided by relatives if the disease is connected with disability, etc.[300]

Disability is often linked with social stigmatization. Stigmatization has its basis in symbolic interactionism—the study of how norms and values are reproduced in our everyday interaction, shaping the proper field of behaviors and skills which are supposed to be followed by the members of a community so that flexibility and desired functioning are achieved. The reduplication of these norms imprinted in the bodies of people with special needs leads to a feeling of a separated actual identity in distinction to a virtual identity which is compatible with community standards. This phenomenon is described as "sticky environments", while the process of negotiation of the discomfort of others by disabled people, placing themselves in a struggle of improvement, individual accomplishments, and self-care, so that the gap between "normal" and "stigmatized" is reduced, is given the term "hidden labor". Medical intervention should not be seen only as an attempt to alleviate the pain of disabled people. We must reconsider if it follows the dominant norms of always attaining a body close to the "normal", and thus contributes to

---

[298]   George L. Engel, "The Need for a New Medical Model: A Challenge for Biomedicine," *Science*, vol. 196, no. 4286 (2016): 29–136.

[299]   Cf. Laurence Foss, The End of Modern Medicine Biomedical Science under a Microscope (New York: State University of New York Press, Albany, 2008).

[300]   Greenhalgh Trisha, Hurwitz Brian,"Why Study Narrative?," *BMJ* (1999): 318–48.

even more social stigmatization. Welfare practices, such as institutions helping disabled people, or offices encouraging work, are not another excuse or a way of legitimating the humanistic façade of the society. The new turn in medical reasoning as described above may help by prioritizing the patient and his subjective experience and reverse this conception of the "diseased body" unfinished in its attempt to reach the "normal body".[301]

Aging is conceived predominantly as individual loss and decline over time, something that is inevitable, personally experienced, and, in a way, universal. Chronological age is used in demographics to describe the percentage of a population which belongs to this irreversible state. Beyond statistics, "aged bodies" are also socially constructed. The discourse encompasses issues like the replacement of the "older working bodies" with new and more capable ones, the management of the health problems associated with physical decline, both by elders' families and the state, and, finally, the changes in our approach to aging if we consider the new technologies and welfare and health care programs addressed to older people.[302] Elders are encouraged to follow a balanced lifestyle, to remain healthy, active, and productive, and thus contribute to the society's well-being as long as they can. This is a project for "active" or "successful" aging, aiming for not only the self-sufficiency of elders but for the disposition of less funding and effort for welfare policies.[303]

The use of robots for elders with mobility problems or dementia raises questions about the different roles of the caregiver, the care receiver, and robots in care praxis. Can the human-machine interaction supplement the embodying experience created by the nurse when he touches or lifts the patient and the oral communication and thus interaction and socialization, which may also include games or songs for maintaining the verbal capacity of elders? Is the interaction between the nurse and the patient an interplay between two living bodies, and thus more profound, while robots can provide only more relational autonomy to the patient

---

[301] Janice McLaughlin, "The Medical Reshaping of Disabled Bodies as a Response to Stigma and a Route to Normality," *Medical Humanities*, no. 43 (2016): 244–50.

[302] A.L Crampton, "Global Aging as Life Course Experience: Results from Ethnographic Research in Ghana and the U.S.," *Innovation in Aging*, no. 1 (2017): 478–478.

[303] Elana D. Buch, "Anthropology of Aging and Care," *Annual Review of Anthropology*, no. 44 (2015): 277–93.

(actions which are linked to the affordances of the agent's environment)?[304]

6.5 Sexual Bodies

Structuralist and post-structuralist feminist theory moved beyond the conceptions of classical feminist theory which mainly deals with the prioritization of masculinity over femininity and the subsequent oppression of women. Sexual bodies are approached through language and the forms that they can take, revealing possible patriarchal narratives, literature, and mythology by analyzing maternal or feminine archetypes, and lately, if we consider the works of Judith Butler, the body has already been shaped in discourses; therefore "biological sex" does not serve as the concrete basis in which gender identity can be grounded.

The sexual body may have a material (biological) reality as itself, but our understanding is always mediated through pre-structured discourses. The notion of *gender performativity* refers to a stylized repertoire of actions which accompany the various performances of gender. Butler proposes that, by adopting gender performances different from the dominant ones, we do not exactly question the process of gender identity construction, since the agents cannot completely change pre-structured discourses (we operate as gendered subjects, in a gendered system), but *gender trouble* starts when we have a failure in the repetition of such actions. A de-formity, or a parodic repetition, can cause a phantasmic effect on the attributing identity which is concretely constructed. An intersexed or hermaphroditic body, for example, may follow this kind of "deformity" and does not fit into the accepted gendered/sexed binary of the *natural* body, thus challenging the whole *natural* binary system.[305]

This breaking of the natural binary system can be expanded to more dis-embodying conceptions of corporeal physicality. Katherine Hayles argues that western thought strives towards an erasure of embodiment and a conception of consciousness as disembodied information. The psychical body in a "posthuman" is just a substrate in which thought and information are attached; thus, the biological embodiment can only be seen as something happening accidentally in history and not as an inevi-

---

[304]   Jaana Parviainen and Jari Pirhonen, "Vulnerable Bodies in Human–Robot Interactions: Embodiment as Ethical Issue in Robot Care for the Elderly," *Transformations Issue*, no. 27 (2017).

[305]   Kathryn Conrad, "Surveillance, Gender and the Virtual Body in the Information Age," *Surveillance & Society*, no. 6 (2009): 380–87.

tability of life. The "posthuman", according to Hayles, concerns the possibilities which information technologies provide. Humans may develop
symbiotic relationships with machines or may be replaced, but there is a
limit in the articulation of humans and intelligent machines, as far as they
remain remarkably different in their embodiments. She follows a dialectical scheme of pattern/randomness which is applied in complex systems.
In this method the meaning is not pre-fabricated; the origin does not act
to ground signification. Complex systems evolve toward an open future
which is characterized by contingency and unpredictability.[306]

Donna Haraway, in her *Cyborg Manifesto*, presents at least three
breakpoints in our transition from the binary relations of man/woman,
mind/body, and nature/culture to more polysemous fusions, uncertain
boundaries, and the marginal space in which the cyborg (as the fusion of
organism and machine) arises. The first concerns the breaking of the
boundary between the human and the animal. Language, the use of tools,
and social behavior cannot define in a persuasive way the limit between
the human and the animal; the cyborg enters the mythical narrative exactly at this point when the above limit is surpassed. The second is the distinction between the human and the machine becoming blurred in the late
20th century. Machines become more and more animated, leaving aside
the classical mind/body and natural/artificial dualisms that defined the
distinctions between humans and machines. The last has to do with the
immateriality of the modern microelectronic devices which are almost
everywhere; they are clean and lightweight because they function with
signals and electromagnetic waves. The cyborg is seen by Haraway as a
figuration of both imagination and reality, structuring any possibility of
historical transformation. It is an entity which belongs to a post-gender
world; it has no linkage with bisexuality, pre-oedipal symbiosis, or unal-
ienated labor, and it has no origin. It is partial, ironic, intimate, and perverted, promoting opposition and utopia, and it is also without inno-
cence.[307]

The theoretical assumptions briefly analyzed above help us to better understand issues like the new forms of sexual interaction in cyber-
environments, as well as the phenomenon of sexual intercourse between
humans and robots or, better, nonhuman entities. Cyber-environments, as
presented in a section of *Virtual Bodies*, provide various ways to either

---

[306] Cf. N. Katherine Hales, *How We Became Posthuman: Virtual Bodies in Cybernetics,
Literature,,and Informatics* (Chicago: The University of Chicago Press, 1990).
[307] Cf. Donna Jeanne Haraway, *Cyborg Manifesto* (Victoria, British Columbia: Camas
Books, 2018).

project or reshape our virtual selves. These selves or—in some cases—avatars are maybe close to Hayles and her analysis of human and intelligent machine augmentation furthermore, flexible virtual environments can be considered as following a dialectical scheme relative to a complex system, that of unpredictability and contingency, since we can transform into a man, a woman, an animal, a human with an animal head, etc. The variability of our sexual representations, as well the newly-emerged field of erotic relationships between humans and non-human entities, can direct our attention to what Haraway defines as the fusion between an organism and a machine or, more specifically, the post-gender world of the cyborg. Beyond the existential and ontological questions which may arise, new (cyber)feminist approaches accuse the dominant patriarchal orientation of sex robots, since in most cases they address the masculine population and both their appearance and voice programming follows aesthetic standards and "the proper" behavior patterns during the interaction cultivated by men.

6.6 Transhuman Bodies

The term *transhumanism* originally comes from the British biologist Julian Huxley, mainly in his *New Bottles for New Wine*, as a unified theory of evolutionary monism. It is a term which stands against religious beliefs, placing man as transcending himself by realizing possibilities of and for his human nature. However, certain philosophies and myths from antiquity (the Saga of Gilgamesh, ancient Greek mythology, Aryanism) and from the Renaissance onwards (Nicolas de Condorcet calls for human perfection with the application of science and techniques, Friedrich Nietzsche presents a philosophy of the Overman, and Charles Darwin describes the origin of species) were determinant for the encapsulation of the term.[308]

There are also anthropological perspectives on the issue of transhumanism; one of the most well-known is that of Andy Clark. He emphasizes the integration of material technologies in the constitution and the evolution of individuals, a conception of the human species as *species technica*. In his "Re-Inventing Ourselves: The Plasticity of Embodiment, Sensing, and Mind", he describes an individual who is capable of incorporating prosthetics and tools that thereby become parts of itself.

---

[308]   Gilbert Hottois, *Philosophie et ideologies trans/posthumanistes* (Paris: VRIN, 2017), 24–48.

This process of prosthesis also engages our cognitive and emotional capacities; it expands in all of our systems. He gives a totally embodied conception of this augmentation in which the mind is under this formation; they are not immaterial entities, not incarnated without a body, but are embodied minds-brains-bodies. To sum up his evolutionary account, he tells us that the human evolved and managed to use tools; these tools now become parts of our inner bodies.[309]

Transhumanism has as a central point not only well-being and general good health, but the possible triumph against aging and physical death, through which we can extract valuable questions such as: the identity and the continuity of the self; ethical questions such as the immorality of a possible immortality; social questions, such as demographics and social relations between privileged persons with enhancements and those without; and—finally—more philosophical questions like the comprehension of functionalism and natural binary systems. Concerning the scientific background of that idea, there are some discrete theoretical points that can be posed. First, there is the image of rejuvenation of the individual who makes use of biomedical and biotechnological methods (targeted intervention in cells with biochemical additives), mainly following the ideas of Aubrey de Grey and Dave Gobel.[310] The second is that of electronic technologies, cybernetics, robotics, etc. which can replace biological organs, and give us the image of the cyborg. Last, there is combination of the two categories at a molecular or sub-molecular level.[311]

Rosi Braidotti criticizes the anthropocentric and anthropomorphic conception of the *person*, which privileges humans over other non-human living entities. This critique does not abandon the idea of a cumulative terrestrial evolution. She calls us to rethink human life (*zoe,* in her words) as a complex ensemble of functions, relations, and processes of a system of evolution which goes in parallel with other technological systems. These systems are characterized by auto-organization, auto-poiesis, and interdependence. It is a conception in which the subject is decentered, multiple, relational, and nomadic, following the philosophy of French post-structuralism (Derrida, Deleuze, etc.).[312]

---

[309]   Ibid., 85–86.
[310]   Aubrey de Grey and Dave Gobel promote the idea of eternal life and are involved in various institutions of cryonics, i.e., the refrigeration of a dead human body with the hope of its preservation and regeneration.
[311]   Ibid., 112–13.
[312]   Ibid., 237–39.

To briefly expound the views on technological singularity, we look at the analyses of Vernor Vinge, Ray Kurzweil, and Nick Bostrom. The first—best-known for his works in literature (science fiction)—in his "The Coming Technological Singularity, How to Survive in Post-Human Era" (1993), gives us an evolutionist account in which technological superintelligence will supersede and marginalize humans. This can be achieved either straightforwardly by technological advancements like artificial intelligence, computer networks, etc., which are capable of an intelligence which is superior compared to the human, or with the amplification of the intellectual capacities of human brains with the cooperation of machines, creating hybrids with advanced cognitive functions. It is a view in which this kingdom of superintelligence will emerge autonomously and remain inaccessible to human reason.

Kurzweil, in his *The Singularity is Near*, follows a scheme in which singularity goes in parallel with paradigmatic changes in our technological know-how. We have had some singular moments in which our limited knowledge has been broadened and has permitted us to obtain a view beyond the past restrictive context. The final stage of this series of evolutionary singular moments will be the technological singularity which will signify the end of biological evolution. There will be a post-singularity era in which there will be no distinction between humans and machines or between physical and virtual reality.

Bostrom, mainly in his *Superintelligence: Paths, Dangers, Strategies*, speculates on the current research in various fields like artificial intelligence (AI), brain scanning that can create digital simulations of the brain (neuromorphic simulations), the enhancement and augmentation of individuals by the use of biotechnology and the interfaces of brain/machine that give us the notion of the cyborg, and the "take off" of superintelligence as a form of superior interconnection between machines which will place the internet in a primitive stage. Superintelligence is differentiated from classical AI to the extent that it can also imitate human intelligence capacities like consciousness, judgment, autonomy, and sensibility. After the last feature, the psychological dimensions that this form of technology can take, he exposes the possible danger of this achievement, like the hegemony it may itself take or be taken by the state or states that can release and control such technology, and asks if it can itself become a singleton as a unique global authority of decision-making pursuing its interests. He makes a distinction between instrumental scopes and final scopes concerning the will of superintelligence on the basis that no intelligent entity without a final scope can preserve its own continuity and identity. Finally, he proposes three forms of control for that technology: first, the existence of a red button which can stop the function of the system if it exceeds certain limits (e.g., domination of humans); second, a "boxing" technique with which specially designed algorithms can break the information input of this kind of superintelligence, especially if expands to the psychical world; and third—and most important and difficult—moral education after the establishment of superintelligence. On what kind of values, norms, and ethical systems should we base it? In any case this technology should attain a general scope so that it will be used for the "good" of humanity and for what humanity really wants.[313]

Conclusions

In this chapter, our main assumption was that technological changes and new digital environments of the information society affect our embodiment in discrete fields. We described six different categories of bodies and revealed the particularity of each case without claiming that there is no overlapping between them. In the first section of *Bodily Governance*, we tried to reveal the gradual changes in the methods of controlling our bodies. Classical sociology and political philosophy were the basis for unfolding this idea. We saw how religious and ethical codes regulating behaviors and evaluating bodily actions were transformed into methods of surveillance, collection of personal and biometric data, and tracking of internet and medical records which stand over and beyond our bodies, shaping a field of an almost deity-like omnipresent impersonal authority; the transition from *panopticon* models to the current *post-panopticon* gives the essence of this important shift. We considered how all these issues affect our social relations in various aspects. For example, how do we conceive of the notion of the citizen, at least as it has been posed after the French and American revolutions, in the spirit of enlightenment, in which freedom, self-realization, justice, and secularism shaped the ideals of the modern liberal state and democracy? How was this made clear in our analysis and which arguments did we use to succeed? Our first argument was that the ethical codes described by Weber, Elias, etc. from the Renaissance onwards have passed to the mentality of the modern state (raison d'etat); this is the classical analysis of Foucault describing

---

[313]   Ibid., 247–274.

biopower (anatomo-politics, when it comes to the techniques of subjugation over the self, such as the care of the self and biopolitics, when biopowerpasses to the population; it is encapsulated by terms like mortality, morbidity, long living), and governmentality (specific calculation of the government), as the dogma of "let them live, or let them die". We proceeded in our argumentation, following Foucault again as we referred to the changes in the European penal system and the forms of discipline and punishment, as well as certain forms of hospitalization, mainly those of psychiatric illnesses, reflecting the social and cultural dimension of madness (in the prism of Foucault's *History of Madness*) in an instrumental way and constructed types such as the monster, the incorrigible, and the masturbator, and placed the patients as abnormal, which still continues in the modern state.[314] Are these interventions forms of bare life such as Agamben poses in his conception of biopolitics? Is this an approach to life that passes from the old Roman empire and the *homo sacer* as someone who could be killed without his killer having any legal consequences, to the Jews in the camps as second category citizens without political rights in the sorrow of the Holocaust, up to the current images of the children in Rwanda suffering from hunger, waiting for the humanistic response of privileged Western people, or the economic immigrants at the ports of Italy jam-packed in modern camps submitted to a new "state of exception"?[315] Continuing our analysis of the new status of the citizen, we focused on the concept of Bauman's liquid modernity and the distinction with heavy modernity. According to Bauman, in heavy modernity, the possibility of totalitarianism was always apparent. In the prevailing Fordist factory routine moves and bureaucracy reduced identities and social interaction to nothingness. In liquid modernity, the process of individuation substitutes the classical notion of the citizen. The citizen now becomes a person without concern for the collective well-being. In this process citizens (persons) are members of a cast which continuously performs tasks.[316] People no longer re-embed themselves in a society as, for example, members of a stable social class, but are constantly on the move, with no end to re-embedding, like musical chairs. There is no option to escape individuation; you just participate in the game.

---

[314]   Cf. Michel Foucault, *Les Anormaux, cours au college de France 1974–1975* (Paris: Gallimard, Seuil, 1999).

[315]   Cf. Giorgio Agamben, *Homo Sacer* (Stanford, Calif.: Stanford University Press, 1998).

[316]   Zygmunt Bauman, *Liquid Modernity* (Cambridge: Polity Press, 2000), 118–25.

We then argued that the body is under a process of continuous transformation. This was made clear in our analysis by describing cases such as classical and 3D-printed organ transplantations, prosthetics, and plastic surgeries. These interventions challenge the limits of our bodies and provide the possibility of reshaping and mutilation. As for transplantations, we claimed that there are ethical and ontological dilemmas, while in prosthetics we focused more on how our embodied actions and *our being in the world* are affected. Finally, plastic surgery not only brings changes in appearance but also alters our embodying experience of the world. A phenomenological approach can be helpful to reveal how these changes can be seen. We can make the distinction between bodies (*Körper*) and lived-bodies (*Lieb*). The lived-body is to feel one's body as one's own body. This is more like a sensation. Husserl speaks of a double sensation; when we touch, the tangible thing emerges, the hand as itself is essential for the tactile perception. The hand separates from the mere body and becomes part of the lived body. The truth (as perceived by the hand) is a truth for the body as a whole. For Heidegger the being of the lived body (*Leibsein*) reveals itself in its embodying (*Leiben*). Embodiment is a mode of being for the body; through this mode we understand that the lived body participates in our subjective perception in distinction with the objectivity of the corporeality when we approach something foreign.[317] Finally, from Merleau-Ponty we can grasp at least two things: first, that our basic level of perceptual experience is the *Gestalt*, as the whole figure against intermediate and contextual aspects of the perceived world as phenomenon, which is not eliminated from a complete account; and, second, that perception transcends itself towards a determinate object in itself, leading to an objective interpretation of the body as something close to kinesthetic awareness and pre-conscious systems of an experienced self (body-schema).

Virtual technologies have an impact on embodying and disembodying experiences. We referred to the technologies used for immersion in virtual spaces in order to make clear what kind of bodily splits may occur. Furthermore, we proceeded with our analysis on the ways avatars socialize, communicate, and interact in digital platforms. We thereby emphasized the issue of how our identity is formed in virtual environments, something that can be seen through the various options

---

[317] Andreas Brenner, "The Lived-Body and the Dignity of Human Beings," in *A Companion to Phenomenology and Existentialism,* ed. Hubert L. Dreyfus, Mark A. Wrathall (New Jersey: Blackwell Publishing, 2006), 478–88.

which the digital platforms provide to project ourselves that either permit us to stay in connection with our inner selves or create the essence of a bodily split between our physical and virtual bodies. Our considerations on medical bodies revolved around the human-based models of medical reasoning and their attempt to criticize the dominant biomedical model which conceives of the patient as a "diseased" body and not as an active agent. We also emphasized that the phenomenon of stigmatization of people with special needs has to be seen in the spectrum of biases created by normative values and beliefs which affect medical praxis and the public welfare system. We also made considerations on the social construction of aging and the questions arising from the interaction of elders with robots and machines used in their care.

In the subsequent section of sexual bodies, our main emphasis was to illuminate the breaking of the "natural" binary systems of thought, mainly after structuralism and post-structuralism. In order to conceive of this breaking, we decided to analyze critical notions such as *gender performativity* and the post-humanist approaches that speak for the domination of information and the possibilities that can provide. This breaking was made apparent from the ideas that support a fusion of a machine and an organism—namely a cyborg.

Finally, as for the last category, *transhuman bodies*, we should concentrate a little bit more on one of their aspects, which is the possible surpassing of death. If we follow Heidegger, this would be another possibility, but, in his existentialist philosophy, death is our ownmost possibility—the way through which we can ascribe a meaning to our Being. If we imagine an immortal human being, could he place himself in a certain horizon of time and thus have a *Dasein* (when he really lives authentically)—a unity of the past-present-future conceiving worldtime? Can such a human live historically?

Conclusions

As we wrote in the introduction, our goal was to point out, from a philosophical perspective, certain aspects of medical practices correlated to the spectrum of biological and social sciences in a society that we have called post-consumerist. How have we tried to reach this particular goal? First, we had to define this kind of society. As we have to a great extent analyzed, the current form of our society is characterized by information knowledge and high technology, although there are changes centered on the form of consumption, which turns into post-consumption; therefore, we called this form of society post-consumerist. In order to clarify these changes, we started from classical political philosophy and social science. We first approached the role that libido plays, which, according to Lyotard, reformulates the forms of exchange as unconditional investment without equivalences. This unconditional investment can be seen in relation with medical philosophy to what Bauman calls fitness, this fragile state in liquid modernity through which the subject always tries to reach a certain point of well-being, but without measurable means, as, for example, the fact of elevated temperature shown by a thermometer when we are feverish. Fitness is the breaking of all norms, the capacity that a flexible body has to possess in order to escape from mundane everyday life. Bauman also claims that the contemporary form of health adopts these characteristics, since we are always trying to be vigilant, to be aware of a possible health problem. As for capital investment, it can be exemplified by all these healthy diets, and by various supplements available even in a local pharmacy, which aim to promote general good health. It can also be exemplified by the overabundance of specialized medical magazines, sites and social media pages, which are devoted to medical issues. Another main point that we posed, again following Lyotard, was that in postmodernity we cannot really subscribe to the great narratives of modernity; what really is the status of therapy today, due to the fact that beyond classical medicine, people turn to alternative medical solutions such as acupuncture, aromatherapy, art therapy, ayurvedic medicine, etc.?[318]

If we follow Baudrillard and his claim that we consume messages and signs rather than commodities, all under a simulation and in a reality

---

[318]   David Låg Tomasi, *Medical Philosophy A Philosophical Analysis of Patient Self-Perception in Diagnostics and Therapy.* (Stuttgart: Ibidem Press, 2016), 171-72.

of hyperreality, we can understand how post-consumers conceive of health care services in their immediacy—through their mass advertising, usually presenting a well-organized and calm hospital environment with patients who smile in relief from their suffering, or even more in various melodramatic TV shows presenting emergency or hard-to-diagnose cases and doctors always capable of resolving them. Finally, Gungov, broadening the conception of Bauman's underclass, claims that the subject today has become an abstract statistical unit which is under various forms of conversions, of real-semblances that can remain real for almost all practical purposes. This statistical view of the self is given in our analysis with the form of real-sembling identity called **trace**. This real-sembling identity has at least three characteristics. First, it participates in various forms of conversions; following the analysis of Gungov, the subject can be investor, voter, protester, taxpayer, or mortgage payer. Second, the subject participates in various predetermined discourses, e.g., social, cultural, political, etc., in its real life. Third, this kind of discourse also takes place in the cyberworld, where in most cases the element of proximity does not exist. So, we can speak for a split identity through which the subject is always seen in a mediated way, without the possibility to form authentic intersubjective relationships. This can be seen after the explosion of Big Data in medicine and biological sciences that either concern data from an over-quantified patient, received from wearable devices which calculate vital parameters, or by the electronic health records of hospitals and we may also consider the data derived from medical research. Furthermore, the patient is someone who can share his personal experience in a digital network community, possibly under the veil of anonymity and by providing faulty information that may be misleading for the other members of the community. But the most serious form of medical manipulation is not that of anonymous patients but that of policymakers and stakeholders that collect and manage all this information from the digitally engaged patients. So, the patient may feel proximity, narrating and sharing his subjective experience of his medical condition, but the next pharmaceutical campaign or advertisement is given in terms of non-proximal and impersonal personality relations, following the trend of a personalized medical intervention. We should declare that, in any case, we do not take into account the major benefits of so-called personalized medicine here; our aim is only to describe how this trend can be used for the commoditization of the patient. But what could be the practicality of a patient as a statistical unit, in the political field, for example?

At the very start of the covid-19 pandemic, when its progress was apparent through the high death toll and the statistical epidemiological models of that time, how did the EU and the European Central Bank, decide to allocate such a large amount of funds for the management of the sanitary crisis (achieving something reasonable while also taking measures for the relief of the debt crisis in the euro zone)?[319] We could also remember the mass civil protests in Belgrade[320] under the veil of various conspiracy theories against the imposed lockdown measures from the government. In this case, abstract statistical units (as possible victims of the pandemic) turn into anti-government protesters almost without any aspiration for a consciousness that could reach a Hegelian Absolute Knowing. However, many things have also changed during the pandemic. Many public opinion-makers who are not necessarily doctors, biologists, or health scientists started to spread their worldviews and conspiracy theories regarding the pandemic, propose alternatives, and speak about a medical and political dictatorship that will control us by the use of microchips and 5G networks.[321] How could we forget the No. 1 tennis player in the world, Novak Djokovic, refusing to be vaccinated, having troubles with the Australian authorities, and not being issued a visa so as to be able to participate in the Australian Open?[322] We should pause here and assert that during extreme conditions like the covid-19 pandemic, there are always voices that push the overall debate to extremes. Although these voices are extremely dangerous for public health and overall social well-being, we should tolerate them, and the scientific and philosophical community should be ready to reply with strong arguments against them. Tolerance of and respect for differences will always be a pillar of the liberal state, rather than the authoritarian imposition of a single view, when it comes to politics and even more when the state in cooperation with medical authorities and stakeholders tries to impose any kind of measure or claim absolute truth. We should not forget that many scien-

---

[319]   Please see: Nicole Scholz, Angelos Delivorias and Marianna Pari, "What can the EU do to alleviate the impact of the coronavirus crisis?" *European Parliamentary Research Service* in: https://www.europarl.europa.eu/RegData/etudes/BRIE/2020/649338/EPRS_BRI(2020)649338_EN.pdf

[320]   Guy de Launey, "Coronavirus: Belgrade protesters storm Serb parliament over curfew", BBC, July 8 2020, https://www.bbc.com/news/world-europe-53332225, last accessed, 25 December, 2020.

[321]   Mark Lynas, COVID: "Top 10 current conspiracy therories," Alliance for Science, April 2020, https://allianceforscience.cornell.edu/blog/2020/04/covid-top-10-current-conspiracy-theories/, last accessed January 28, 2022.

[322]   "Novak Djokovic: Australia cancels top tennis player's visa", BBC, January 6, 22, https://www.bbc.com/news/world-australia-59889522, last accessed January 28, 22.

tists were threatened or abused for discussing covid-19 survey finds—
something even more threatening to democracy.[323]

Our second objective from the scope of moral philosophy was to
describe the various mechanisms through which manipulation and disinformation are spread by the elites. This could help us to see how this
real-sembling identity we called **trace** is involved within intersubjective
relationships, both in a non-mediated and mediated way, how these relationships in relation with proximity lead to the subject's subjugation by
the elites, and if there is some kind of alternative based on the notions of
arbitrariness and the Hegelian topsy-turvy world, the last permits us to
better clarify how, in the post-cosumerist society, there is always a possibility for the existence of double realities—the one that is, let it say, the
things as themselves, as they are, and the other, a real-sembling reality
which coexists and is here for all the kind of conversions that we analyzed. This is no way of returning to German Idealism and to ideas that
could seem as outdated. It should be seen more as a tool which helps us
to better clarify some phenomena, rather than a form of another one
mechanistic scheme. We started from a classical phenomenological and
hermeneutical analysis—here, Heidegger, Levinas, and Gadamer were
the main sources—to deepen the various ways through which the subjects perceive time, history, tradition, language, and the Other. We be-
lieve that this general introduction was necessary to provide a more concrete basis on which an intersubjective relationship is based, either connected with the meaning of Being, or as a fusion between horizons, or—
finally—as an asymmetrical ethical relationship. In order to clarify these,
we described the relation between those who belong to the center (elites)
and those who belong on the periphery (statistical units). We claimed
that statistical units are interconnected through their proximity, and with
the center through their **trace** and real-semblance. The definitive point
was that it is the non-proximal relation between the center and the periphery which stands as the factor of the imposition of dominance of the
elites over the periphery; here, classical phenomenology, hermeneutics,
and structural analysis were the main methods of describing this kind of
relation. We also claimed that the subjects (statistical units), in order to
surpass the general signification posed by the elites, contextualizing a
normative or correct field of authority, should proceed to a process of

---

[323]   "Scientists abused and threatened for discussing Covid, global survey finds", The
Guardian, November 21, https://www.theguardian.com/world/2021/oct/13/scientists-a
bused-and-threatened-for-discussing-covid-global-survey-finds, last accessed January
28, 22.

mutual glaring. Here we also would like to reemphasize the notion of performativity of action as described in our analysis. Beyond its axiological value, it tries to reveal the fact that the subject (at least) as approached from structuralism onwards is decentered, saturated. It always participates in predetermined discourses that are constructed by social, political, and religious norms. The performativity of the action transfers the attention to the performing act and the results that it may have. Consequently, if a patient (or a doctor) participates in these discourses and the patient presents views on his condition that may have (for example, a religiously constructed discourse). If, in the case of a mental illness, the patient claims that his condition is the result of a possession by an evil spirit, the doctor should be evaluated based on his efficacy of diagnosis and healing. Furthermore, if we deepen this relation, this action, in order to be ethical, it should be mutually glared. Doctor and patient, in their one-to-one relation, first should see out of a general signifier, which places the correct field of authority on the subject's normativity, as posed by elites—e.g., that this person may be deviant, dangerous, abnormal, etc.

Continuing our analysis in a more general vein—a possible topos of mutual glaring could be their relation with time. If we follow Heidegger and his analysis, the fundamental ontological care of the hermeneutics of Being as itself is connected with the inquiry about the temporality (*Zeitlichkeit*) of Being.[324] Therefore, if the patient can have the subjective feeling of his illness as a rupture in time—as something restrictive—and thus cannot make possible projections into the future, the doctor—even if he makes use of Bayesian statistics to make a prediction of a future event—definitely contemplates in time. The time of prognosis should be seen as a fusion of the temporality of the doctor and patient. Furthermore, when a doctor passes from Big Data to smart data, from a patient in general to this patient, he separates himself from the objective time of Big Data; additionally he separates himself from a possible diagnosis (conceived of as general signifier that has been produced by a process of data correlation) and his time, the time of the action, becomes time in relation with his patient by grasping the signs, symptoms, clinical facts, and even subjective feelings of the patient, and so manages to make a signification that includes the patient in an active way; he understands how the patient progresses in time, either towards recovery or towards exacerbation.

---

[324]   Martin Heidegger, *Being and Time* (Oxford: Blackwell, 1962), 402.

In the third chapter, we strove towards a philosophy of biology and neuroscience or a better classical philosophy of science. We started by analyzing computational neuroscience, a form of neuroscience that represents our brain as networks of neurons. We tried to reveal why this view of neuroscience could be conceived of as subjective and reductive, since it equates the mind with the brain and does not account very much for the social and cultural factors that can better encapsulate the notion of the mind. Furthermore, it is incapable of approaching higher complex phenomena linked to human behavior, such as reproduction, self-repair, and adaptation to new environments. We also tried to exhibit its strong connection with artificial intelligence programs, known as connectionist. These programs are capable of imitating human imagination since they can compute, combine in other words, to produce schemata. So, in a manner, to threaten human imagination. We strove towards metaphysics, psychoanalysis, and speculative poetics, in parallel with John Ashbery's "Self-Portrait in a Convex Mirror", to propose that human imagination, in distinction to the imagination of non-human entities like machines, produces not only schemata but also noemata. We then presented the theory of mirror neurons, which can be seen as neuroscientific theory—incorporating elements of an intersubjective approach since it refers to the grasping of intentions and the emotions of others and to phenomena like empathy and learning. Through the latter, it refers to human evolution, also encompassing some elements of sociality and culture. Although there are valuable findings from this theory, we also explored the serious critique against it, mainly proposed by Gregory Hickok, so that mirror neuron theory would not be seen as evidence-supportive but as complementary in providing a basis in the phenomenon of "mutual understanding". Additionally, we tried to find parallels between mirror neuron theory and phenomenology and heurmaneutics, mainly those of Husserl, Scheler, Merleau-Ponty and Gadamer. We also focused on cases in which being acts in opposition to an extra-signified context, as a response to an extra-being, cases that attain exteriority through the overcoming of restrictive limits, the passing from one restrictive context to another-Dehors (eschatological exteriorizing), through the (o)thereness, following the **traces** of the (o)ther non-linear human being. In medical praxis, this happens in chronic diseases or diseases with a therapy which is unknown; in these cases, the *medicus* may break with protocol and test experimental therapies, usually first on cell cultures then through genetic mechanics on a molecular base, then to animals, but only after the randomization on humans. Consequently, the doctor has to see beyond the curtain of the theater to touch supersensibility, and—even if does is not always involve a breaking of an epistemological maxim—the doctor balances and measures the benefits of such a decision. This is quite important since, when we speak of chronic diseases, the patient can possibly be in a position where he/she cannot make projections. He/she simply lives in a condition which subjectively is taken as a rupture of his/her well-being and an inability to recover or to establish new rules in his/her daily life and environment. Then appears the role of the Doctor. Let's say the chronic disease or a disease with an unknown treatment is another case of a restrictive context—Dehors in our case. This Dehors is the incomprehensible and the impossible to treat, but this incomprehensible is something different for the patient and the doctor. The first cannot anymore be an active agent; he/she simply surrenders to the hopes provided by the doctor and the progress of medical science. It is my anymore (as a patient) as a human being, and my very being towards science in general. The doctor gradually has to collect all the signs to look carefully at all the symptoms and clinical data, and finally all the possible findings, from evidence-based medicine and possible new treatments and surpass this restrictive Dehors. The Dehors is also the patient's nomore as a human being and not only the lack of knowledge and incapability of the doctor to act and perform this or that treatment. We speak for a relationship (one to one) in which both participants simply both can't. However, the doctor is the one who is not only morally obliged to decide but also to act. The time of the action is the time of the surpassing of the restrictive Dehors; it is not something incomprehensible anymore but is a possible new beneficial treatment, a new protocol. In another case, imagine a doctor who treats a patient in a vegetative state. In this case, the restrictive context is more serious; it is a more restrictive Dehors. The patient cannot simply react, but his/her life relies upon the mechanical support of the ventilator, the monitor, etc. The doctor always has to measure in these cases, and his/her action is an action in the grey zone between life and death. Levinas here says that I am not only responsible for my death but the death of the Other as well. However, the patient in the best-case scenario is the Third; the doctor from another point of view is the one who tries in all possible ways to preserve the patient in a vegetative state in life, and in some cases, of course, where the inevitable is always apparent, to overcome any restriction and to have a first conscious breath after a coma. This is the reason that we passed from poetry and poetics to this eschatological exteriorizing. Human imagination cannot in any case be just a scheme, a correlate of a computational system, or a connectionist unit. Life and death are not just two parameters of a powerful computer that could propose this or that treatment; they are two parameters that remind us of our mortality and futility. However, human imagination as translated to medical thinking and science in our case is not exactly the triumph over death, but rather this very remembering that—even in cases where we have absolutely nothing in our mind (in our case, concrete medical knowledge)—we are capable of overcoming any restrictive context. This very actuality was already there and is another word for human hope. All these considerations lead us to rethink, from an epistemological perspective, the limits of medical science in general and the fact that medicine and philosophy of medicine can create puzzles.

Another major assumption that we tried to reveal here, in this chapter devoted to classical epistemology and theory of science, is how medicine and medical philosophy create puzzles and problems which simultaneously define their theoretical and practical boundaries as a response to the debate of whether philosophy of medicine can be a separate field. In order to achieve this, we explored two different approaches, the dominant biomedical model and the second more human-based model. The two models have different foundations and different worldviews; this is why we chose to refer to Thomas Kuhn and his theory of paradigmatic changes: to reveal how medicine (and the philosophy of medicine) can create puzzles, propose models which reflect their particular worldviews, and also define the subject matter of the field, placing its practical and theoretical boundaries. The biomedical or objective model of medical reasoning has as its ultimate raison d'être, substance matter. It holds a materialist or physicalistic view of the body, which is reduced to a diseased entity, through which physicians obtain objective clinical data so as they can proceed to medical interventions. The humanistic or subjective form of reasoning has at its core a holistic or dualistic metaphysical view, since it seeks to explore the subjective experience of the patient and how he symbolically interacts with his social and cultural environment. The call for the humanization of medicine starts from the claim that the doctor may adopt a distanced role and that there is not much concern for the particularity of the patient and the way he experiences his condition—for example, how he lives sentiments of pain, suffering, and anxiety and how they contribute to the progression of his problem and healing. Furthermore, there are external factors, social, cultural, internal, etc. In the humanistic model, the patient is not approached as a diseased body, but as an active agent with a particular subjectivity; thus, the doctor-patient relationship turns from the interpretation of data (based in statistics and evidence-based medicine) which aims at the patient's safety and substantiation of knowledge into an intersubjective active communication which passes to the sphere of the patient's subjective experience and concerns. Hence, according to Eric Cassell, physicians have a narrow understanding of objectivity while subjectivity prevails; e.g., when someone has fever, the objective state is the evaluation of the temperature with the thermometer, but the feverishness is something subjective. Cassell gives five rules for substantiating medical knowledge: the values that a society has regarding health and illness, the general goals of the medical care, the personal values of the doctor, the individual values of the patient, and the values of the system as a whole. George L. Engel accuses the biomedical model of a conceptualization of disease as deviation from the norm of the measurable, and contends that the social, physiological, and behavioral dimensions of the illness are not a part of its approach. Laurence Foss emphasizes the role of information in conjunction with the brain and the body; with his memes as replication information units, he theorizes how anorexia nervosa is linked with the social norms of "you are never thin enough", and how this is expressed in the metabolism. Lastly, the narrative model is the storytelling of the subjective feelings of the patient; this storytelling may be a basis for sharing temporalities as we described above. Furthermore, we explored the social and ethical dimension of medical practice as seen in the doctor-patient relationship, emphasizing the changes that have occurred in the relationship in the information age. We started from classical conceptualizations of models describing the physician-patient relationship, to pass to the patient as a well-informed (post)consumer who demands control of his condition and information about the offered services as well as methods of not wasting time in the digital age and a doctor who tries not to lose his "powers" as the expert who knows, reformulating his medical practice according to the demands of the patients interacting with cyber-environments.

   Continuing with the chapter in which we described the impact of Big Data on medicine, our aim was to expose its applicability to medicine and the role that it may play in diagnostics, preventive medicine, and therapeutics, here epistemology was our concern one more time. We also exposed the methods and models with which it is generated and how knowledge can be acquired through it. Beyond its practical scope, in our concluding remarks we would like to re-emphasize the epistemological problems that can occur from the generation and management of Big Data. These problems may arise from its nature, such as the curse of dimensionality which concerns optimization in Big Data sets, or the missing values that may bias conclusions. Additionally, we focused on the problems revolving around causality in the models representing biological functions. Furthermore, we approached the limits of the randomized control trials in the form of a total skepticism but in a form of reconsideration since they seem to be the gold standard for contemporary medicine. We posed issues like the prior knowledge that is needed for the implementation of a protocol of a trial and the problems that may occur because of unbalanced results. One of our major concerns was what happens with the fourth paradigmatic change in science which shapes a data-intensive conception of science based on an obscure empiricism and which replaces causation with correlation and claims that that is enough. All these brought us to the need to emphasize the idea of patient safety, as proposed by Gungov, and the use of abductive reasoning, over the inductive and deductive, which is contextual and relies on experience and decision strategy. Additionally, since Big Data is generated in various domains of Science we chose to approach it through the prism of an integrative object, as proposed by Schmid and Mambrini Doudet, which acts in relation with other objects; it invites a dynamic of knowledge and is not synthesizable. Finally, we proposed a scheme which uses the theory of Levinas and his primacy of ethics and Derrida's practico-ethics, while in our perception we gave emphasis to our main assumptions such as the glaring and the ethics of performativity of action and arbitrariness. We closed the chapter by referring to the debate between naturalism and normativism. Our basic aim in this case was to admit that there are difficulties in the definition of health and disease. This definition becomes more complicated after the extreme quantification of health in the age of Big Data and the double sense that health adopts as being objective and in parallel contributing to the creation of normative claims and evaluations like the "average patient" or the "statistically deviant". Furthermore, from the middle of the 20th century, there were voices accusing biomedicine of adopting an extreme naturalist view, neglecting to incorporate the social dimension of phenomena no longer conceived of as diseases, like alcoholism, masturbation, homosexuality, and menopause. So we compared the naturalist view of Boorse, who speaks for a value-free and objective definition of health, the moderate normativism of the holism of Nordenfelt, the concept of biological normativity proposed by Ganguilhem, and, finally, the hybridist account of Stegenga, who holds that there is both a causal and normative basis of disease and emphasizes the role of medical efficacy.

As for our last chapter, we would like to focus a little bit more on the aspects which are mainly related to medicine. First, we saw how the collection of biometric data can shape the ideal of the citizen without genetic defects and far from the risk of an unhealthy lifestyle, such as alcohol consumption, as criteria to obtain so-called neurological and biological citizenship; this could be related to what Giorgio Agamben calls bare life. Furthermore, concerning organ donations and transplantations, how do they alter our subjective experience of our bodily image? Is the role of medicine challenged, since this passes from a purpose of care to a rally to advance the human race? In continuation, with organ transplantation, will 3D-printed biomaterials solve the problem of organ trafficking or facilitate the receiver to have immunosuppressive therapy which is essential after the operation? What happens with testing and the possible problems of irreversibility? As for prosthetics, is there a possibility of losing our conceptual links with the world if we consider the various phantom phenomena that appear, and consequently the way we understand our being in the world? Additionally, we would like to focus our attention on the stigmatization of disability, based on symbolic interactionism and the hidden labor to which disabled people are submitted in order to meet the norms and the social standards of a healthy body. We then focus on the new conceptions of aging and the continuous encouragement of elders to follow a balanced diet and a healthy lifestyle. In the case of the use of robots in the care of elders, mainly with mobility problems or dementia, do they really challenge the usual human interaction between two living bodies—i.e., the elder and the nurse? Finally, the theories of transhumanism challenge the limits of our physicality, of our finitude, and of possibly ascribing a meaning to our existence; is the triumph over death really what we aspire to in our lives? Do we look to dominate nature even more and, if we fuse with the machine, could this solve the problems of decline, of demographics, and even equality with the Other within society?

This book was written during the covid-19 pandemic. Its goal was not to be another philosophical analysis of the coronavirus, and this is the reason that we did not insist very much on that. It is a book which, by chance, was written during these two very difficult years for humanity. What we should maintain is that we are human beings with names, families, friends, etc. I do not even refer to us as citizens, parents, scientists, philosophers, etc. In any case, we are not simple statistical units, even though, at around 8:00 p.m. every day, we learn that a considerable number of people have been infected or died. It is a book that aims to propose that we are not simply the **They,** the **Das Man.** We should not stop thinking, rethinking, and speculating on the new forms of the information and disinformation society we reside in, and that we have called post-consumerist. If we claim that our identities are split and have given it the name trace, we can always—in our authentic intersubjective interaction, either as simple human beings or as exemplified in the doctor-patient relationship—overcome obstacles, act, and, of course, love each other and tolerate. This tolerance is the other name for the metaphysical violence of coexisting. If this awful experience of the pandemic comes to an end, we should be united, humane, and charitable.

Bibliography

Adorno, Teodor. *Negative Dialectics*. New York: Seabury Press, 1973.

Aerts et.al., Diderick. *World Views from Fragmentation to Integration*. Ebook. Clément VandAlexanderRiegler 2007. https://www.researchgate.net/public ation/244529051_Worldviews_From_Fragmentation_to_Integration.

Agamben, Gorgio. *Homo Sacer*. Stanford: Stanford University Press, 1998.

Agostinho, Daniela. "Big Data, Time and the Archive." *symploke* 24, no. 1 (2016): 435–45.

Anagnostopoulos, A, Katsafadou, A. I., Pierros, V., Kontopodis, E., Fthenakis, G. C., Arsenos, G. Tsangaris. "Milk of Greek sheep and goat breeds; characterization by means of proteomics." *Journal of Proteomics*, no. 147 (2016): 76–84.

Anagnostopoulos, Athanasios, Katsafadou Angeliki, Pierros Vasileios, Kontopodis Evangelos, George C Fthenakis, Arsenos George, Ch Karkabounas Spyridon, Tzora Athina , Skoufos Ioannis, and Th Tsangaris George. "Dataset of Milk Whey Proteins of Three Indigenous Greek Sheep Breeds." *Data in Brief Elsevier Inc*, no. 8 (2016): 877–80.

Anderson, Chris. "The end of theory: The data deluge makes the scientific method obsolete." *Wired*, June 23, 2008, http://www.wired.com/science/discove ries/magazine/16-07/pb_theory, last accessed, December 24, 2020.

Atherton, J.C. "The pathogenesis of Helicobacter pylori-induced gastro-duodenal diseases." *Annu Rev Pathol*, no. 1 (2006): 63-96.

Alizadeh, MB, Eisen RE Davis, C Ma, IS, Lossos, A. Rosenwald, et al., "Distinct types of diffuse large B-cell lymphoma identified by gene expression profiling." *Nature*, no. 11 (2000): 403-503.

Arendt, Hannah. *The Human Condition*. Chicago: The University of Chicago Press, 1988.

Ball, Kristie, Laura Maria Di Domenico, and Daniel Nunan. "Big Data Surveillance and the Body-Subject."*Body & Society*, no.22 (2016): 58-81.

Barberouss, Anouk.,. Franceschelli Sara, C. Imbert. Computer simulations as experiments." *Synthese*, no. 169 (2009): 557–74.

Barberousse, A., M. Vorms "About the Empirical Warrants of Computer-Based Scientific Knowledge.", *Synthese*, no. 191 (2014):3595–620.

Bataille, George. *Erotism:Death And Sensuality*. Los Angeles: City Lights, 1986.

Bates, Laura. 2017. "Opinion | The Trouble With Sex Robots." *Nytimes.Com*, July 7, 2017, 2020. https://www.nytimes.com/2017/07/17/opinion/sex-robo ts-consent.html?mcubz=0, last accessed, January 25, 2020.

Baudrillard, Jean. *Symbolic Exchange and Death*, trans. Iain Hamilton Grant. London: Sage, 1993.

Baudrillard, Jean. *The Consumer Society, Myths and Structures*. London: Sage, 1998.

Bernard, Claude. *Introduction à la médecine expérimentale, considérations expérimentales spéciales aux êtres vivants.* Paris: Livre de poche, 1988.

Biocca, Frank, and Levy Mark. *Communication Applications of Virtual Reality.* Hillsdale: Lawrence Erlbaum Associates, 2015.

Birke, Lynda. "Soma Kai Viologia." In *Viokoinonikoties Ta Oria Tou Somatos Diepistimonikes Prosegisis.*Athens:Nisos, 2014.

Bogard, William. *The Simulation of Surveillance: Hypercontrol in Telematic Societies.* New York: Cambridge University Press, 2016.

Brenner, Andreas. The Lived-Body and the Dignity of Human Beings." In *A Companion to Phenomenology and Existentialism* ed. Hubert L. Dreyfus, Mark A. Wrathall, 478–88. New Jersey: Blackwell Publishing, 2006.

Buch, Elana. "Anthropology of Aging and Care." *Annual Review of Anthropology*, no. 44 (2015): 277–93.

Bauman, Zygmunt. *Liquid Modernity.* London: Polity Press, 2000.

Bauman, Zygmunt. *Consuming Life.* Cambridge: Polity Press, 2007.

Bauman, Zygmunt and David Lyon. *Liquid Surveillance a Conversation.* Cambridge: Polity Press, 2016.

Broad, C. D. *The Mind and Its Place in Nature.* London: Kegan Paul, Trench, Trubner & Co., 1925.

Caplan, A.L. "Does the Philosophy of Medicine Exist?" *Theoretical Medicine*, no. 13 (1992): 67–77.

Capurro, Rafael. "Medicine in The Information Society and Knowledge", Keynote at the European Summit for Clinical Nanomedicine and Targeted Medicine (CLINAM), Bassel Switzerland, June 23–26, 2013, http://www.capurro.de/Medicine2_0.html, last accessed, December 20, 2020.

Casile, Antonio, Vittorio Caggiano, and Pier Francesco Ferrari. "The Mirror Neuron System: A Fresh View."*The Neuroscientist: A Review Journal Bringing Neurobiology, Neurology and Psychiatry*, no.17 (2011): 524–38.

Cartwright, Nancy. "Are RCTs the Gold Standard." *Biosocieties*, no. 2 (2008): 11–20.

Cartwright, Nancy. "What Are Randomised Controlled Trials Good For?" *Philosophical Studies*, no. 147 (2010): 59–70.

Cassell, Eric. *The Nature of Suffering and The Goals of Medicine.* New York: Oxford University Press, 2014.

Chazard, Emmanuel. "Réutilisation et fouille de données massives de santé produites en routine au cours du soin". HdR diss., LilleUniversité, 2016.

Clauson, K. H Polen, M, Kamel Boulos, J Dzenogiannis. "Scope, completeness, and accuracy of drug information in Wikipedia." *Ann Pharmakometer*, no. 42 (2008): 1814–21.

Clemnet, J. "Google, Amazon, Facebook, Apple, and Microsoft (GAFAM) - statistics & facts." Statista.com, accessed, January 25, 2020, https://www.statista.com/topics/4213/google-apple-facebook-amazon-and-microsoft-gafam/, Last accessed, December 20, 2020.

Clegg, Joshua W., and Brent D. Slife. "Epistemology And The Hither Side: A Levinasian Account Of Relational Knowing." *European Journal of Psychotherapy & Counselling*, no. 7 (2005): 65–76.

Cohen-Levinas, Danielle, and Marc Crépon. *Levinas-Derrida*. Paris: Hermann, 2014.

Conard, Kathryn. "Surveillance, Gender and the Virtual Body in the Information Age." *Surveillance & Society*, no. 6 (2009): 380-87.

Contrearas, Brian. "Bezos, Zuckerberg and other Big Tech chiefs answer to Congress on antitrust concerns." *Los Angeles Times*, July 29, 2020, https://www.latimes.com/politics/story/2020-07-29/congress-to-grill-tech-industry-chiefs, last accessed, December 20, 2020.

Crampton, A.L. "GLOBAL AGING AS LIFE COURSE EXPERIENCE: RESULTS FROM ETHNOGRAPHIC RESEARCH IN GHANA AND THE U.S." *Innovation in Aging* no. 1 (2017): 478–478.

Cunningham, Thomas V. "Objectivity, Scientific City, and the Dualist Epistemology of Medicine." In *Classification, Disease and Evidence, History, 1 Philosophy and Theory of the Life Sciences*. Springer Science + Business Media Dordrecht, 2001.

Cullen, Bernard. "Philosophy of existence 3, Merleau-Ponty." In *Twentieth-Century Continental Philosophy*, ed. Richard Kearney. London: Routledge, 1994.

Davis, Ann. "The Body as Password." *Wired*, January 7, 1997, https://www.wired.com/1997/07/biometrics-, last accessed, January 25, 2020.

Deaton, August. "Instruments, Randomization and Learning about Development." *Journal of Economic Literature*, no. 48 (2010): 424–455.

Deleuze , Gilles and Félix Guattari. *Anti-Oedipus: Capitalism and Schizophrenia*, translated by Robert Hurley, preface by Michel Foucault, introduction by Mark Seem. Mineapolis, Minessota: University of Minessota Press, 1984.

Deleuze, Gilles. *Logic of Sense*, Translated by Constantin V. Boundas. London: The Athlone Press, 1990.

Derrida, Jacques. *Writing and Difference*. London: Routledge Classics, 1978.

De Launey, Guy. "Coronavirus: Belgrade protesters storm Serb parliament over curfew", *BBC*, July 8 2020, https://www.bbc.com/news/world-europe-5333 2225.

De Vries, E.N., H.A. Prins, R.M. Crolla, A.J. den Outer, G. van Andel, S.H. van Helden, et al., "Effect of a comprehensive surgical safety system on patient outcomes." *New England Journal of Medicine*, no. 363 (2010) : 1928–37.

Dictionnaire des sciences médicales, par une société de médecins et de chirurgiens, édition de Panchoucke, Paris, 1819, article « Nosographie ».

Dimitrova, Maria. *Sociality and Justice: Toward Social Phenomenology*. Stuttgart: ibidem Press, 2016.

Dimitrova, Maria. "Personal Identity: From Belonging Toward Responsibility." *Sofia Philosophical Review*, vol. IV, no. 2, 2010.

Dinov, Ivo. "Methodological challenges and analytic opportunities for modeling and interpreting Big Healthcare Data," *GigaSience*, no. 5 (2001).

Docherty, Thomas. "Postmodernist theory. In *Twentieth-Century Continental Philosophy*, ed. Richard Kearny. London: Routledge, 1994.

Dreyfus, Hubert. *On The Internet*. New York: Routledge, 2008.

Dufva, T. and M. Dufva. "Grasping the future of the digital society." *Futures*, no. 107 (2019): 17–28.

Engel, George. "The Need for a New Medical Model: A Challenge for Biomedicine." *Science*, no. 4286, (1971) : 129–136.

Espinasse, B., P. Bellot. "Introduction au Big Data—Opportunités, stockage et analyse des mégadonnées", *Technologies De L'information | Technologies Logicielles Architectures* Des Systèmes (2001).

Esteva, A., B. Kuprel, R. Novoa, J. Ko, S. Swetter, H. Blau,S Thrun. "*Dermatologist-level classification of skin cancer with deep neural networks.*" *Nature*, no. 542 (2017): 115–118.

Evidence-Based Medicine Working Group. "Evidence-based medicine: a new approach to teaching the practice of medicine." *JAMA*, no. 4 (1992): 2420–5.

Ewing, GW. "The limitations of big data in healthcare." *MOJ Proteomics Bioinform,* no. 5 (2017): 40–43.

Fajans, S.S G.I., Bell, K.S. Polonsky. "Molecular mechanisms and clinical pathophysiology of maturity-onset diabetes of the young." *N Engl J Med*, no. 345 (2001): 971–980.

Fayyad, Usama, Gregory Piatetsky-Shapiro, and Padhraic Smyth. "From Data Mining to Knowledge Discovery in Database." *AI Magazine*, no. 17 (1996): 37.

Foss, Laurence. *The End of Modern Medicine Biomedical Science Under a Microscope*. New York: State University of New York Press, Albany, 2008.

Foucault, Michel. *The History of Sexuality. Vol. 1*. London: Penguin Books, 1998.

Foucault, Michel. *Les Anormaux, Cours au College de France 1974–1975*. Paris: Gallimard, Seuil, 1999.

Fu, A.Q., D.P. Genereux, R. Stoger, C.D. Laird, M. Stephens. "Statistical inference of transmission fidelity of DNA methylation patterns over somatic cell divisions in mammals." *Ann Appl Stat*, no. 4 (2010): 871–92.

Gadamer, Hans-Georg. "Culture and the World." In Hans-Georg Gadamer, *Praise of Theory: Speeches and Essays*, translated by Chris Dawson. Yale University, New Haven, 1998.

Gadamer, Hans –Georg. *Truth and Method*. Michigan: Seabury Press, 1977.

Gallese, V., L. Fandiga, L. Fogassi, G. Rizzolati. "Action recognition in the premotor cortex." *Brain*, no. 119 (1996): 593–609.

Gallese, V.A. Goldman. "Mirror Neurons and the simulation theory of mind-reading." *Opinion*, no. 2 (1998): 493–501.

Gallese Keysers, Rizzolatti. "A unifying view of the basis of social cognition." *Trends in cognitive sciences*, no. 8 (2001): 396–403.

Gallese, V. "The shared manifold hypothesis: From mirror neurons to empathy." In E. *Between ourselves: Second-person issues in the study of consciousness*, ed. Thompson, 33–50.

Gillespie, Tarleton. "The Relevance of Algorithms." In *Media Technologies: Essays on communication, materiality, and society*, ed. T. Gillespie, P. J. Boczkowski, and K. A. Foot. Cambridge Mass.: MIT Press, 2014.

Gilbert, Frederic, Cathal D. O'Connell, Tajanka Mladenovska, and Susan Dodds. "Print Me an Organ? Ethical And Regulatory Issues Emerging From 3D Bioprinting in Medicine." *Science and Engineering Ethics*, no. 24 (2017).

Giroux, Elodie. "Philosophie De La Medicine. In *Précis De Philosophie Des Sciences*, ed. Barberousse, Anouk, Denis Bonnay, and Mikaël Cozic. Paris: Vuibert, 2015.

Giroux, Élodie. *Après Canguilhem*. Paris: Presses universitaires de France, 2014.

Giudice, Marco, Manera del Valeria and Christian Keysers. "Programmed to Learn? The Ontogeny of Mirror Neurons." *Developmental Science*, no. 12 (2009): 350–63.

Glick, S.M. "Humanistic medicine in a modern age." *N Engl J Med*, no. 304 (1981): 1036–38.

Godard, Jean Luc. 1965. *Alphaville, Une Étrange Aventure De Lemmy Caution*. Film. France: Chaumiane.

Goodwin, Brian Carey. *How The Leopard Changed Its Spots*. Princeton N.J: Princeton University Press, 2001.

Gratton, Peter, "Jean François Lyotard", *The Stanford Encyclopedia of Philosophy* (Winter 2018 Edition), Edward N. Zalta (ed.), URL = <https://plato.stanford.edu/archives/win2018/entries/lyotard/>.

Greenhalgh, Trisha and Brian Hurwitz. "Why study narrative?" *BMJ*, no. 318 (1999): 48.

Gulshan, V. et al. "Development and validation of a deep learning algorithm for detection of diabetic retinopathy in retinal fundus photographs." *JAMA*, (2016).

Gungov, Alexander. "Real Semblance Flourishing in Post-Consumerist Society." *Sofia Philosophical Review*, vol. VII, no. 2, 2013.

Gungov, Alexander. *Patient Safety: the Relevance of Logic in Medical Care*. Stuttgart: ibidem Press, 2018.

Hales, N. Katherine. How We Became Posthuman: Virtual Bodies in Cybernetics, Literature, and Informatics. Chicago: The University of Chicago Press, 1990.

Haraway, Donna Jeanne. *Cyborg Manifesto*. Victoria, British Columbia: Camas Books, 2018.

Harvey, David. "The new imperialism. Accumulation by disposesion." *Social Register*, no. 40 (2004): 63–67.

Heidegger, Martin. *Being and Time.* Oxford: Blackwell, 1962.

Hey, Anthony J. G, Stewart Tansley, Kristin Michele Tolle. *The Fourth Paradigm*. Redmond, Wash.: Microsoft Research, 2009.

Heyes, Cecilia. "Tinbergen on Mirror Neurons." *Philosophical Transactions of the Royal Society of London. Series B, Biological Sciences*, no. 369 (2014).

Humphrey, P. "The philosophical novelty of computer simulation methods," *Synthese,* no.169 (2008): 615–26.

Huijgen, R, M.N. Vissers, J.C. Defesche, P.J. Lansberg, J.J. Kastelein, and B.A. Hutten. "Familial hypercholesterolemia: Current treatment and advances in management." *Expert Rev.Cardiovasc*, no. 6 (2008): 567-81.

Iacoboni, Marco, Molnar-Szakacs Istvan, Vittorio Gallese, Giovanni Buccino, and John C. Mazziotta. "Grasping the Intentions of Others with One's Own Mirror Neuron Syste." In *PLoS Biology*, no.3 (2004):529–35.

Ingelfinger, FJ. "Medicine: meritorious or meretricious." *Science,* no. 200 (1978): 942–946.

MG, Jaffe, Lee GA, Young JD, Sidney S, Go AS. "Improved blood pressure control associated with a large-scale hypertension program." *JAMA*, no.310 (2016): 699–705.

Jeurgens, C. Threats of the data-flood: An accountability perspective in the era of ubiquitous computing. In F. Smit, A. Glaudemans, & R. Jonker. Archives in Liquid Times, 2016.

Johnston, Adrian, "Jacques Lacan", *The Stanford Encyclopedia of Philosophy* (Fall 2018 Edition), Edward N. Zalta (ed.), URL = <https://plato.stanford.e du/archives/fall2018/entries/lacan/>.

Kitchin, Rob. "Big Data, New Epistemologies and Paradigm Shifts." *Big Data & Society*, (April 2014).

King, M.C, J.H. Marks, J.B. Mandell, and the New York Breast Cancer Study Group. "Breast and ovarian cancer risks due to inherited mutations in BRCA1 and BRCA2." *Science*, no. 302 (2003): 643–46.

Knosel, Michael, Klaus Jung. "Information Value and bias of videos related to orthodontics screened on a video-sharing Web Site." *Angle Orthod*, no. 81 (2011): 532–9.

Lajochere, Jean Patrick. "Role of Big Data in evolution of the medical practice" Bull. Acad. Natle Méd., séance du 6 février, 2018.

Lazer D, Kennedy R, King G, et al. "The parable of Google Flu: Traps in big data analysis." *Science*, no. 334(2016): 434.

"Latin Definition for Emergo." Ladict, last modified January 29, 2020, http://lati n-dictionary.net/definition/19005/emergo-emergere-emersi-emersus

Lee, C H Yoon. "Medical big data: promise and challenges." *Kidney Research and Clinical Practice*, no. 36 (2017):3–11.

Lee, PY, KP. Alexander, BG. Hammill, et al. "Representation of elderly persons and women in published randomized trials of acute coronary syndromes." *JAMA* no. 286 (2001): 708–13.

Levinas, Emmanuel. "Humanism and An-Archy." *Revue Internatinal De La Philosophie,* no. 85 (1968): 65–82.

Levinas, Emmauel. "Meaning and Sense." *Humanisme De L ' Autre Homme,* (1972): 7–63.

Levinas, Emmanuel. Time *and the Other,* trans. Richard. A. Cohen. Duquesne University Press, 1987.

Levinas, Emmanuel. *Entre Nous: On Thinking-of-the-Other,* translated Michael B. Smith and Barbara Harshav. New York: Columbia University Press, 1998.

Lewis, R.J, R.L Wears. "An introduction to the Bayesian analysis of clinical trials." *Annalsof Emergency Medicine,* no. 22(1999):1328–36.

Lyotard, Jean Francois. *Libidinal Economy,* translated by Iain Hamilton Grant. Indianapolis: Indiana University Press, 1993.

Malone, K.E., J.R. Daling, D.R. Doody, L. Hsu, L. Bernstein, R.J. Coates, P.A. Marchbanks, M.S. Simon, J.A. McDonald, S.A. Norman, B.L. Strom, R.T. Burkman, G. Ursin, D. Deapen, L.K.Weiss, S. Folger, J.J. Madeoy, D.M. Friedrichsen, N.M. Suter, M.C. Humphrey, R. Spirtas,and E.A. Ostrander. "Prevalence and predictors of BRCA1 and BRCA2 mutations in apopulation-based study of breast cancer in white and black American women ages 35 to 64 years." *Cancer Res,* no. 66 (2006): 8297-8308.

Marcuse, Herbert. *One-Dimensional Man.* London: Routledge, 2002.

Marcum, James. *Humanizing Modern Medicine: An Introductory Philosophy Of Medicine.* Springer, 2008.

Markie, Peter, "Rationalism vs. Empiricism." *The Stanford Encyclopedia of Philosophy* (Fall 2017 Edition), Edward N. Zalta (ed.), URL=<https://plato.stanford.edu/archives/fall2017/entries/rationalism-empiricism/>.

Manzoni, C. D. Kia, J. Vandrovcova, J Hardy, N Wood, P Lewis,& R Ferrari. "Genome, transcriptome and proteome: the rise of omics data and their integration in biomedical sciences." *Briefings In Bioinformatics,* no. 19 (2016): 286–302.

Martin, Bland Altman Douglas G. "Bayesians and frequentists." *BMJ,* (1998): 317–1151.

Martin, Emily. "Mind-Body Problems." *American Ethnologist,* no. 27 (2000): 569–90.

Mattingly, C. 1998 "In search of the good: narrative reasoning in clinical practice." *MedicaAnthropology Quarterly,* no. 12: 273–97.

McLaughlin, Brian. *The Rise and Fall of British Emergentism.* Beckermann, A., Flohr, H., & Kim, J, 1992.

Mc Partland, James C, Brian Reichow, and Fred R Volkmar. "New Research: Sensitivity and Specificity of Proposed DSM-5 Diagnostic Criteria for Autism Spectrum Disorder." *Journal of the American Academy of Child & Adolescent Psychiatr, no.* 51 (2012): 368–83.

Mayo, DG and A Spanos. *Error and Inference: Recent Exchanges on Experimental Reasoning, Reliability, and the Objectivity and Rationality of Science.* New York, NY: Cambridge University Press, 2010.

MIAMI Trial Research Group. "Long-term prognosis after early intervention with metoprolol in suspected acute myocardial infarction: experiences from the MIAMI Trial." *J Intern Med, no.* 230 (2001): 233–7.

Mill, Jonh Struard. *System of Logic. Ratiocinative and Inductive. Collected Works, Volumes 7 and 8.* Toronto: University of Toronto Press, 1996.

Miguel, Juan Carlos, Angel Cassado del Rio. "GAFAnomy (Google, Amazon, Facebook and Apple): The Big Four and the b-Ecosystem." *Dynamics of Big Internet Industry Groups and Future Trends,* (2016): 127–148.

Médecine pratique de Sydenham. Avec des notes. Ouvrage traduit en français sur la dernière ed. anglaise par M.A.F. Jault Paris 1784 (préface des observations, 1666). Préface de l'auteur.

Merleau-Ponty, Maurice. *Phenomenology of Perception: An Introduction.* London: Routledge, 2011.

Morie, Jacquelyn Ford. "Performing in (Virtual) Spaces: Embodiment and Being in Virtual Environments." *International Journal of Performance Arts and Digital Media, no.* 3 (2006): 123–38.

Munster, Anna. *Materializing New Media.* Hanover, N.H.: Dartmouth College Press, 2012.

Murra, D. "Towards a Phenomenology of the Body in Virtual Reality." *Research in Philosophy and Technology,* (2000): 149–73.

Murphy, Robert. *The Body Silent.* London: J.M. Dent and Sons Ltd, 1997.

Murray E., B. Lo, F Pollack, K. Donelan, J. Catania, M. White, K. Zapert , R Turner, "The impact of health information on the internet on the physician–patient relationship." *Arch Intern Med, no.* 163 (2003): 1727–34.

National Research Council. *Toward Precision Medicine: Building a Knowledge Network for Biomedical Research and a New Taxonomy of Disease.* Washington, DC: The National Academies Press, 2011.

Negri, Antonio, Michael Hardt. *Empire.* Cambridge: Harvard University Press, 2000.

Nishiyama, K., V. Johnson. "Karoshi—Death from Overwork: Occupational Health Consequences of Japanese Production Management." *International Journal of Health Services: Planning, Administration, Evaluation, no.* 27 (1997): 625–41.

Parviainen Jaana, and Jari Pirhonen. "Vulnerable Bodies in Human–Robot Interactions: Embodiment as Ethical Issue in Robot Care for the Elderly." *Transformations Issue, no.* 27 (2017).

Perkins, Jan, and Daniel Wang. "A Comparison of Bayesian and Frequentist Statistics As Applied In A Simple Repeated Measures Example." *Journal of Modern Applied Statistical Methods*, no. 3 (2004).

Peterson, D.C., C. Martin-Gill, F.X. Guyette, A.Z. Tobias, C.E. McCarthy , S.T. Harrington , et al. "Outcomes of medical emergencies on commercial airline flights." *N Engl J Med*, no. 368 (2011): 2075–83.

Pollett, Simon W. John Boscardin, Eduardo Azziz-Baumgartner, Yeny O. Tinoco, Giselle Soto, Candice Romero, Jen Kok, Matthew Biggerstaff, Cecile Viboud, George W. Rutherford. "Evaluating Google Flu Trends in Latin America: Important Lessons for the Next Phase of Digital Disease Detection." *Clinical Infectious Diseases*, no. 64 (2017): 34–41.

Quintin, Jacques. "Organ Transplantation and Meaning of Life: The Quest for Self Fulfilment." *Med Health Care and Philos*, no. 16 (2012): 565–574.

Ratcliffe Matthew, "Phenomenology, Neuroscience, and Intersubjectivity." In *A Companion to Phenomenology and Existentialism*, ed. Hubert Dreyfus and Mark A. Wrathall. London: Blackwell, 2006.

Reed M., J. Huang , R. Brand , I. Graetz , R. Neugebauer , B. Fireman , et al. "Implementation of an outpatient electronic health record and emergency department visits, hospitalizations, and office visits among patients with diabetes." JAMA, no. 310 (2013): 1060-65.

Rizzolati, G. L.Fadiga, V.Gallese, L.Fogassi. "Functional organization of inferior area 6 in the macaque monkey." *Experimental Brain Research*, no. 71(1988): 491–507.

Rom, Hare. *Physical Being*. Oxford: Blackwell ,1991.

Rossello, X, S.J. Pocock, D.G. Julian. "Long-term use of cardiovascular drugs: challenges for research and for patient care." *Journal of the American College of Cardiology*, no. 66 (2015): 1273–85.

Roukos, D.H and E. Briasoulis. "Individualized preventive and therapeutic management of hereditary breast ovarian cancer syndrome." *Nat. Clin. Pract. Oncol.* no. 4 (2001): 578-590.

JC. Atherton. *The pathogenesis of Helicobacter pylori-induced gastro-duodenal diseases*. Annu Rev Pathol., no. 1 (2006): 63–96.

Sackett, D.L, W.M. Rosenberg, J.A. Gray, R.B. Haynes, and W.S. Richardson. "Evidence-Based Medicine: What it Is and What it Isn't," *British Medical Journal*, no. 312 (1996): 71–72.

Scholz, Nicole Angelos Delivorias and Marianna Pari, "Whatcanthe EU doto alleviate theimpact of thecoronavirus crisis?" *European Parliamentary Research Service* in: https://www.europarl.europa.eu/RegData/etudes/BRIE/2 020/649338/EPRS_BRI(2020)649338_EN.pdf

Schmid, Anne-Françoise, and Muriel Mambrini-Doudet. *Épistémologie Générique*. Paris: kime, 2019.

Schubert, Carl Mark C van Langeveld, and Larry A. Donoso. "Innovations in 3D Printing: A 3D Overview from Optics to Organs." *The British Journal of Ophthalmology*, no. 98(2): 159–61.

Sharon, Tamar. "Self-Tracking For Health And The Quantified Self: Re-Articulating Autonomy, Solidarity, And Authenticity In An Age Of Personalized Healthcare." *Philosophy & Technology*, no. 30 (2016): 93–121.

Shilling, Chris. "The Rise Of Body Studies And Embodiment". *Horizons in Humanities and Social Sciences*, no. 1 (2016): 22–46.

Sirota, Chana. "3D Organ Printing". *The Science Journal of the Lander College of Arts and Sciences*, no. 10 (2006).

Stegenga, Jacob. *Medical Nihilism*. Oxford: Oxford University Press, 2018.

Symons, John, and Ramón Alvarado. "Can We Trust Big Data? Applying Philosophy of Science to Software." *Big Data & Society* no. 3 (2016).

Sheridan, Desmond J., and Desmond G. Desmond G. "Achievements And Limitations Of Evidence-Based Medicine." *Journal of the American College of Cardiology*, no. 2 (2001).

Switankowsky, I. "Dualism and its importance for medicine." *Theoretical Medicine,* no. 21 (2001): 567–80.

Tandon, R W Gaebel, RBarch M Bustillo, J.Gur, RE Heckers, S. Carpenter, W. "Definition and description of schizophrenia in the DSM-5." *Schizophrenia Research* (October, 2013).

"The Cambridge Analytica Files", *The Guardian*, https://www.theguardian.com/news/series/cambridge-analytica-files, last accessed, December 20, 2020.

Tomasi, David Låg. *Medical Philsophy a Philosophical Analysis of Pateint Self-Perception in Diagnostics and Therapy*. Stuttgart: Ibidem Press, 2016.

Trakle, Sherry. *Alone Together*. New York: Basic Books, a member of the Perseus Books Group, 2012.

Van Spall, H.G, A. Toren, A. Kiss, et al. "Eligibility criteria of randomized controlled trials published inhigh-impact general medical journals: a systematic sampling review." *JAMA*, no. 297 (2007): 1233–40.

Verene Donald Phillip. *Speculative Philosophy,* Lanham: Maryland, Lexicom books, 2009,

Wald, Hedy S. Catherine, E.Dube, David C. Anthony. "Untangling the Web— The impact of Internet use on health care and the physician–patient relationship." *Patient Education and Counseling*, no. 63 (2006): 24–28.

Weisbord, SD JB Soule, PL Kimmel. "Poison on line—acute renal failure caused by oil of wormwood purchased through the Internet." *NEJM* no. (1997): 825–27.

Yuasa T, S Urakami, S Yamamoto , J Yonese , K Nakano , M Kodaira, et al. "Tumor size is a potential predictor of response to tyrosine kinase inhibitors in renal cell cancer." *Urology*, no. 77 (2001): 831–35.

Appendix

IN RELATION WITH CHAPTER 2

Conceptual Diagram
Contextualization

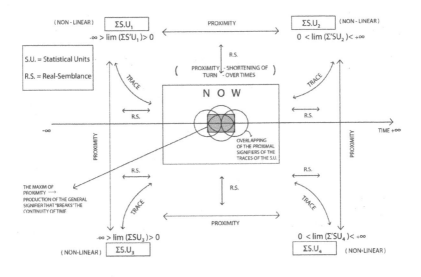

Conceptual Diagram
Decontextualization

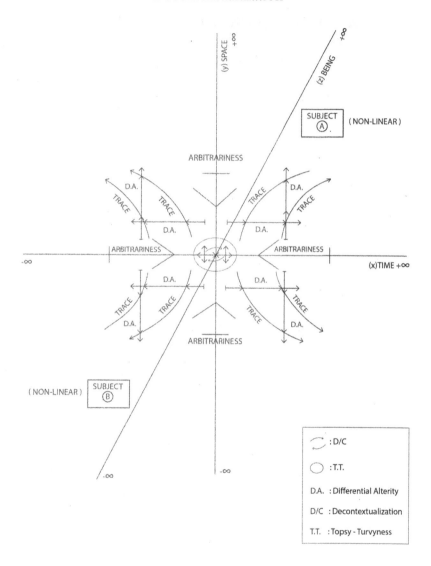

Self-relation (BUT WITH SENSING)

What is to be = what is [prior] to be like =
to be like this (progress of a general signification)

(o) -thereness (overcoming of the lack)

What is to be=what is [prior] to be a-like to be like ≠ (IN SUBLATION) =
what is other than this a-like =a sublatednon-reciprocal/non-univocal

reciprocal / univocal
transcending of the : to be like (general signification) =
practical self-comprehending modality

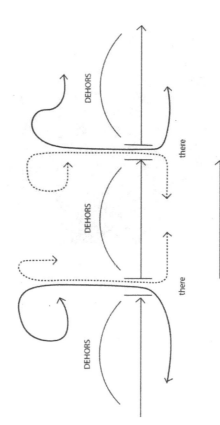

DEHORS

DEHORS

DEHORS

there

there

Conditioning = Space+time+Signification+immanence

A Possible Formalization: Meaning and Sense in the Post-consumerist Society / transcending of the : To be like (General Signification)

IN RELATION WITH CHAPTER 3

Guggenheim New York

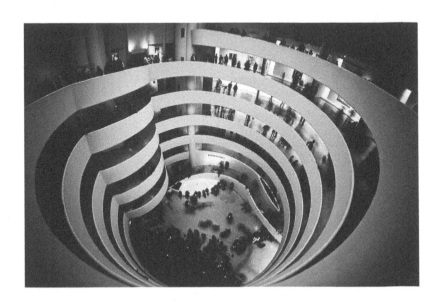

Guggenheim Bilbao

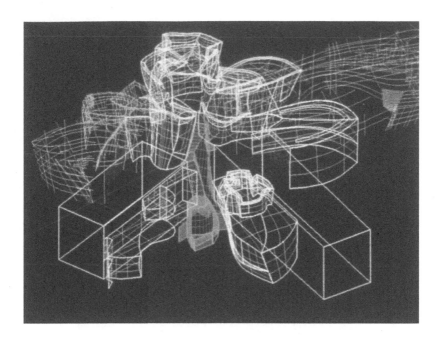

Conceptual
DiagramClinamen

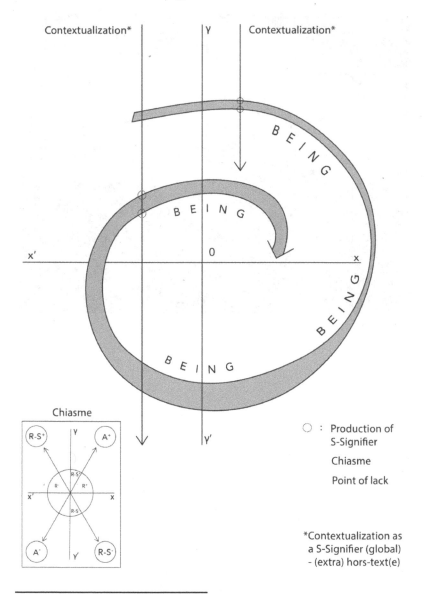

i   Alexander Gungov, Patient Safety: *The Relevance of Logic in Medical Care* (Stuttgart: Ibidem Press, 2018), 67–68.